MW00614186

Counting the Dead

Counting the Dead

The epidemiology of skeletal populations

TONY WALDRON
Institute of Archaeology, London, UK

JOHN WILEY & SONS
Chichester • New York • Brisbane • Toronto • Singapore

Copyright © 1994 by John Wiley & Sons Ltd,
Baffins Lane, Chichester,
West Sussex PO19 1UD, England

Telephone   National   Chichester (0243) 779777
International   +44 243 779777

All rights reserved.

No part of this book may be reproduced by any means,
or transmitted, or translated into a machine language
without the written permission of the publisher.

Other Wiley Editorial Offices

John Wiley & Sons, Inc., 605 Third Avenue,
New York, NY 10158-0012, USA

Jacaranda Wiley Ltd, 33 Park Road, Milton,
Queensland 4064, Australia

John Wiley & Sons (Canada) Ltd, 22 Worcester Road,
Rexdale, Ontario M9W 1L1, Canada

John Wiley & Sons (SEA) Pte Ltd, 37 Jalan Pemimpin #05-04,
Block B, Union Industrial Building, Singapore 2057

Library of Congress Cataloging-in-Publication Data

Waldron, T. (Tony)
     Counting the dead : the epidemiology of skeletal populations / by
Tony Waldron.
          p.   cm.
     Includes bibliographical references and index.
     ISBN 0-471-95138-2
     1. Paleopathology.   I. Title.
     [DNLM: 1. Paleopathology. 2. Bone and Bones—pathology. QZ 11.5
W167c 1994]
     R134.8.W35   1994
     616.07—dc20
     DNLM/DLC
     for Library of Congress   94–8477
                                                                    CIP

British Library Cataloguing in Publication Data

A catalogue record for this book is available from the British Library

ISBN 0-471-95138-2

Typeset in 11/13pt Palatino from author's disks by Production Technology Department,
John Wiley & Sons Ltd, Chichester
Printed and bound in Great Britain by Biddles, Guildford, Surrey

*I would like to dedicate this book
to the memory of my mother*

Contents

Preface

I wrote this book in order to illustrate the use of epidemiological methods in palaeopathology and to encourage their use more widely than is presently the case. I hope that it will be informative and instructive and that it might even be entertaining in parts.

I have received a lot of encouragement from many sources during the preparation and writing of the book. I am grateful to all my colleagues and friends who have withstood my constant droning on about epidemiology at meetings, both formal and informal, and who have responded with ideas and suggestions which have been helpful, useful, and sometimes ignored. My special thanks go to my wife Gillian who has always been my most ardent critic and who has weathered the storm which surrounded this book's gestation with equanimity and good humour, as well as correcting both grammar and sense. I would like to have the courage, as Austin Bradford Hill did in the preface to the seventh edition (1961) of his *Principles of Statistics* to say of those who had proffered advice to him, sincerely to trust that the reader would hold them largely responsible for any faults which remain; but I can't quite do it. If readers do find faults, I hope they will write to me in case there is an opportunity in the future to put these right; I would also be pleased to hear from any readers who actually like the book.

Finally, I must mention the staff at John Wiley & Sons who have been an absolute pleasure to work with and I would like to formally express my thanks to them for making the transition from disk to printed page so painless.

Tony Waldron
London, 1994

Introduction

I came into palaeopathology, like many others I imagine, by a roundabout route. My background had included—in varying amounts—biochemistry, anatomy, epidemiology, toxicology, occupational medicine and medical history. I first became interested in bones after I had carried out some historical research on the history of lead poisoning and came upon Gilfillan's notion that the fall of Rome had its origin in this disease.[1] While it was evident that the Romans had exposed themselves considerably to lead, it was equally clear that to ascribe their demise to this single cause was too simplistic. Nevertheless, it seemed that it might be possible to make some assessment of their lead exposure—and that of other populations—from a consideration of the lead levels in their bones since the hard tissues contain more than 90% of the total body burden of lead. Accordingly my colleagues and I analysed several hundred bone samples and stopped only when we realised that we were not taking lead uptake from the soil sufficiently into account; when we made some investigations of the amount of lead which the bones might be absorbing post mortem, it seemed that we had probably spent far too much time on this trail and abandoned it.[2]

During the sampling of the many skeletons which were included in our studies, I could not but become interested in the diseases which were present and it seemed to me that it would be much more fruitful to begin to look at the prevalence of disease in past populations and study how this might have changed through time. Almost as soon as I began seriously to study skeletons,

however, a number of epidemiological problems were encountered which did not seem to me to have been considered
greatly in what I was able to read of other workers in this area. As
in so much of epidemiology, the problems were principally with
denominators but there were a number of other questions, not
least amongst them the problem of diagnosing disease in bones.

The result of the deliberations over the years form the basis of this
small book. Many of the ideas have been tested out at meetings,
large and small, and in informal conversations with colleagues.
The book begins with a consideration of the development of
palaeopathology and where it fits; is it a branch of medicine, of
anthropology or of medical history? My own conviction is that it
is best considered as a branch of medical history since it must
surely have as its principal aim the delineation of patterns of
disease in the past and may legitimately use any information
which is reasonable to accomplish that aim. When dealing with
skeletons or other human remains, however, the tools of epidemiology must be applied since the objects of the study constitute a
population—or at least a sample of it—however flawed.

The difficulties encountered in palaeoepidemiology begin with
the populations under study and these are considered in the
second chapter. It is probably true to say that, faced with the
samples with which the palaeopathologist has to work, any modern epidemiologist would quickly find something else to occupy
his time as there is almost nothing about them which would satisfy
his exacting requirements. If one insists on working with skeletons
or any other human remains, however, there is no hope of anything better than the archaeologist can retrieve and one must
perforce use what there is despite its imperfections, the most
serious of which is the almost total lack of randomness. Knowing
the imperfections in the material may help to temper the claims
made for it; and that is the theme of this chapter.

To the non-medical person it often comes as a surprise to learn
how imprecise the process of diagnosis is in medicine and how
full of fashionable vagaries. The tyro in palaeopathology assumes
that he will be able to ascertain the cause of each abnormality—
large or small—and may be disillusioned to be told by some of
those more experienced that the chances of actually achieving this

are slender to say the least. Shopping round, however, he will soon find that there is no shortage of those who *will* profess to be able to offer an exact diagnosis for each and every lesion and they may even feel confident of the ways in which the various conditions seen owe their existence to the life style or occupation of the deceased and, conversely, how they will have modified that life. It is the earnest intention of Chapter 3 to dispel such notions and recommend an altogether more diffident line, one which I suggest is much more in accord with our potential to cull real information from our forebears.

Chapters 4–6 are the heart of the matter and contain suggestions firstly on how the frequency of disease in skeletal populations should be determined, differentiating rates which may legitimately be calculated (prevalence and proportional morbidity) from those which cannot (incidence and all others commonly used in modern epidemiology). There follows a chapter which discusses how the prevalence of disease may be compared between studies using either odds ratios or standardisation. A method by which the common odds ratio can be calculated is described. The two principal methods of standardisation also are described and recommendations are given as to which of these is the most appropriate to use in palaeoepidemiology.

The final objective of this group of chapters is to outline some methods which can be used to carry out what are often referred to as analytical studies in epidemiology, the most important of which is the case control study. This is not a textbook of epidemiology; these are already plentiful—too plentiful some might say— and mention is made of those which I have found most useful or the most pleasurable to read. Statistics and mathematics have been kept scarce and simple and even the most extreme 'numerophobe' should find nothing to produce anxiety or panic. My intention has been only to suggest paths through this rather troublesome terrain; those who wish for more detailed information on the topography will need larger scale maps.

There follows a short chapter which should be considered as a suggested guide to 'best practice'. In it I have tried to summarise the suggestions made throughout the book and to make a plea for some commonality of method and reporting.

The final chapter deals with occupation, which is of particular interest to me because this is my specialist field in medicine. Many authors have devoted much time to deducing the occupation of those long dead from the imperfections in their bones in the understandable—but ill conceived—attempt to recreate their life style. The only other area of study which has attracted more effort has been the deduction of environmental stress—whatever that is—from the skeleton. Some extraordinary claims have been made about the origins of disease, especially osteoarthritis, in individual skeletons, and in Chapter 8 I show that occupation *cannot* be deduced from lesions in the skeleton. I do not expect that those who wish it otherwise will be persuaded that such is the case, but I do hope to put doubts into the minds of those who are not committed to the notion, so that they will view claims which are made about the activities of our ancestors with a good deal of scepticism. We should, with Francis Bacon, be wary lest 'we ... give out a dream of our imagination for a pattern of the world'.

NOTES

1. S. Gilfillan, Lead poisoning and the fall of Rome, *Journal of Occupational Medicine*, 1965, 7, 53–60.
2. See, for example, H.A. Waldron, Post-mortem absorption of lead by the skeleton, *American Journal of Physical Anthropology*, 1981, 55, 395–8.

1

The Development and Nature of Palaeopathology

Human remains have excited the curiosity and interest of the general public for centuries but their systematic study has been erratic and most often a fringe activity of those whose professional interests were principally directed elsewhere. The first accounts of the studies of fossil bones appeared in the 18th century and Esper is generally given priority for his report on what he considered to be an osteosarcoma in the femur of a cave bear but which was subsequently explained by Mayer in 1854 as a simple fracture.[1] The reports which followed in the 18th and the early part of the 19th centuries by such men as Goldfuss, Cuvier, Clift, von Walther and Schmerling were, in the main, concerned with fossilised animal bones which were turned up by chance from time to time, especially those of cave bears and lions.[2] Human bones began to be studied to any extent only in the wake of three major events. The first was the migration of settlers to the west coast of America when large quantities of Indian remains were encountered; the second was the discovery of fossil hominids in France and Germany; and the third, and perhaps most significant, was the excavation of the cemeteries in Nubia in advance of the construction of the Aswan Dam on the Nile, which produced enormous numbers of skeletons and mummies.[3]

The earliest studies of human remains were given over very largely to the description of isolated pathological abnormalities or conditions and followed very much the medical model current at the time, but it is with these studies that palaeopathology might be said to have its origins.

There are often great anxieties attached to the paternity of new medical disciplines and it has been customary to accord the privilege of fathering palaeopathology to Virchow in consideration of his publication on Neanderthal bones in 1872.[4] Virchow described shortening of an ulna and humerus, which he considered was due to rickets, and osteoarthritis (arthritis deformans) in Neanderthals. The diagnosis of rickets was substantiated much later by Ivanhoe.[5]

Studies in Europe, however, had lagged behind those in America where J.C. Warren and S.G. Morton had produced works on the crania of the mound builders between 1822 and 1839, and began what Jarcho described as a cranial fixation which persisted well into the first half of the present century.[6] Both Warren and Morton described artificial cranial deformation and, in Morton's case, trauma; the first study of disease in ancient human remains in the United States was undertaken almost half a century later by Joseph Jones, whose monograph appeared in 1876.[7] Amongst the conditions which Jones reported in his assemblage was syphilis, and his efforts and those of other early American workers have been well described by Jarcho.[8]

The huge volume of human remains which was uncovered by the archaeologists between about 1880 and 1930 stimulated a great deal of activity in palaeopathology, associated especially with the names of Ruffer, Wood-Jones and Elliot Smith in Britain, Pales in France and Hrdlicka and Moodie in America. Three classic texts appeared in this period, Moodie's *Paleopathology*, the *Paléopathologie et pathologie comparative* of Pales, and Ruffer's volume on the palaeopathology of Egypt.[9] Ruffer's volume was a collection of papers brought together by his widow and published four years after his death at sea during the First World War, with the help of Moodie who acted as editor.[10] This book contains the paper in which Ruffer first used the term palaeopathology, and which he thought he was introducing into the language.[11] Moodie, in his book, pointed to a definition in the *Standard dictionary* of 1895, which was the earliest reference he was able to find and which antedated Ruffer by almost 20 years.[12] There is, however, an even earlier use of the term dating to 1893. Writing in a paper in the *Popular Science Monthly* on the pathology found in some fossil bird bones, Schufeldt, an American physician, suggested it as a term

> under which may be described all diseased or pathological conditions found fossilized in the remains of extinct or fossil animals.

I have been unable to find any use of the term prior to Schufeldt and he probably does deserve the credit for it.[13]

The early palaeopathological studies were largely descriptive, detailing findings in interesting individual cases or groups of cases; this practice has continued to the present day and provides a substantial proportion of all the publications in this field. However, an important new phase in palaeopathology was signalled by the publication of Hooton's study of the Pecos Indians in 1930.[14] In his account of the early history of palaeopathology, Pales described three phases. He considered that palaeopathology

> à traversé trois grandes périodes. Dans la première, de 1774 à 1870 environ, on écrit des essais limités à la pathologie de la faune quarternaire.

> Dans la deuxième, de 1870 à 1900, ce sont surtout les lésions traumatiques humaines et la recherche de l'origine de la syphilis ...[15]

> Dans la troisieme période, de 1900 à nos jours, les auteurs ont orienté leurs recherches vers les maladies infectieuses ...[16]

Roney, writing in 1959, saw Hooton's study as marking the beginning of the fourth stage, that of the palaeoepidemiological study.[17] The importance of Hooton's work was that he treated the assemblage he examined as a population and applied population statistics to his results, reporting prevalence data for some pathological conditions, including osteoarthritis; there was for osteoarthritis of the spine a considerable increase with age, which is entirely to be expected, but no definite trend with sex. The prevalence of this condition in young adults (21–35 years) was 3.03%; in middle-aged skeletons (36–50 years) it was 34.55% while in old skeletons (> 50 years) the figure was 62.12%.[18]

Roney pointed to a number of other studies which had used population statistics to estimate the prevalence of disease or to calculate life expectancies[19] and himself made an important contribution through his account of the pathology in the remains excavated from a site in California, calculating prevalence rates for a number of different conditions.[20] His conclusions would now be viewed with caution in view of the small number of individuals he studied (44 in total; 27 adults) and the very fragmentary nature of the skeletons, both of which would introduce a wide margin of error into his calculations.

Hooton's paper was not to be the start of another fruitful period in palaeopathology; the subject languished from the 1930s onwards (Jarcho actually marked the decline somewhat precisely to the publication of Herbert Williams's last major paper in 1936[21]) and few medical practitioners took much of an interest in it. Indeed the trend seemed to be for archaeologists to select those skeletons which showed obvious signs of disease and find a physician willing to write a report on them for inclusion in a larger body of work to which it was entirely peripheral. When a revival came in the late 1950s and early 1960s, it was brought about largely through the medium of physical anthropology, and palaeopathology was no longer considered a branch of medicine.[22] Angel marks the beginning of this modern period of palaeopathology as having three stimuli: Jarcho's 1965 symposium, the publication of Brothwell and Sandison's *Diseases in antiquity* and the formation of the Paleopathology Association by Aidan Cockburn and others.[23]

There continued to be an epidemiological thread in much of the work which was carried out in the 1960s and 1970s but what might be called the interpretive element was dominant and it has become more influential as the medical input into the subject has tended to become diluted, although contrary to what I seem to be saying, one of the most notable proponents of interpretive palaeopathology, Calvin Wells, was a medical man, for many years a general practitioner in Norfolk.[24]

Of course all data require to be interpreted but the distinguishing mark of scientific interpretation is that ideas are put forward which can afterwards be tested. This is often expressed formally in terms of hypothesis testing although it has to be said that outside the pages of learned journals and grant applications, science tends to proceed in a largely informal way, and the idea of *a* or *the* scientific method is something of a modern myth.[25]

Many of the interpretations given in palaeopathology, however, are expressed without qualification as facts, not opinion, or in a form which is not amenable to testing (and frequently both). Often the premise for the interpretation is wrong or misguided and may not touch anywhere upon modern clinical thought or experience. There is a deep-seated desire to obtain a definitive diagnosis: to determine the exact *cause* of the observed lesion and to discourse on the effects which this disease must have had on the individual. Frequently, an occupation is confidently ascribed to a skeleton on the basis of a pattern of osteoarthritis or hyperostoses, or a graphic account is given of sufferings which would be remarkable if one had a medical history, several years of clinical notes and the results of X-rays and laboratory tests to hand. The performance of some exponents of interpretive palaeopathology is such as to suggest, in Isaiah Berlin's wonderful phrase, that 'their gifts lay in other spheres'.[26]

The urge to provide a good story for one's readers is so tempting as to be well nigh irresistible for many workers in this field and although this may make for better reading than a more factual report it also makes for less rigorous work, it is less intellectually challenging and does not do much to take the discipline beyond the realm of myth and fable.

THE NATURE OF PALAEOPATHOLOGY

The early definitions of palaeopathology placed it very clearly in a medical context by limiting it to the study of disease in fossilised remains. It was not long before it came to apply to more recent remains, however, especially in the United States where to equate pre-history with the pre-Columbian period places it in the very recent past to European eyes. Medical historians also have a considerable interest in palaeopathology, however, since it offers a way objectively to answer some questions about the antiquity of disease, but from their point of view other sources of evidence, such as works of art, may provide additional evidence which, if only indirect information, may nevertheless be useful. Temkin was firmly of the view that the palaeopathologist was 'a medical historian specializing in diseases of ancient man and in the methods appropriate for such study' and he placed palaeopathology as a specialty of the history of medicine.[27] In this, Temkin was confirming the much older assertion of Klebs who wrote in 1917 that palaeopathology was 'historical research because it endeavors to supply data in the evolution of mankind ...'[28] Some later authors have also emphasised a broad definition; Kerley and Bass have written that 'not only skeletal material but disease itself is the subject matter of paleopathology'.[29]

The view taken here is sympathetic to that which sees palaeopathology as fitting most comfortably within the ambit of medical history and that one of the most important tasks for those who practise it is to trace the history of disease in both human and animal populations, studying changes in its frequency and factors which may have affected it. To do this, all kinds of information may legitimately be used, although the remains of those who lived before us are the most significant since they provide the most direct evidence. And since the study of the frequency of disease relies upon the use of epidemiological tools, the purpose of this book is to encourage their use in a more systematic fashion than has generally been the rule to date.

NOTES

1. E.J.C. Esper, *Ausführliche Nachrichten von neuentdeckten Zoolithen unbekannter vierfüssige Thiere*, Nuremberg, 1774. Esper (1742–1810) was professor at Erlangen. F.J.C. Mayer, Über krankhafte Knochen vorweltlicher Thiere, *Nova Acta Leopoldina*, 1854, 24, 673–89. Mayer's work contained a review of the palaeopathological literature in addition to his own description of the lesions found in 24 bones from cave bears and lions.
2. The early history of palaeopathology is described by R.L. Moodie, *Paleopathology*, University of Illinois Press, Urbana, 1923, chapter 1 and H.E. Sigerist, *A history of medicine*, New York, Oxford University Press, volume 1, 1951, pp. 38–65.
3. W.R. Dawson, in his foreword to *Diseases in antiquity* (edited by D.R. Brothwell and A.J. Sandison, Springfield, C.C. Thomas, 1967) says that thirty thousand skeletons and mummies were excavated at this time (pp vii–x).

4. Rudolf Virchow (1821–1902) was the most famous pathologist of his day. He held the first full chair in pathology in Germany (at Würzburg) and subsequently was professor in Berlin. One of his outstanding contributions was to found, with Benno Reinhardt, the *Archiv für Pathologische Anatomie und Physiologie* in 1846, a publication which is still in print.

   Before his note on Neanderthal bones, Virchow had published some observations on cave bears in 1870 but his interest in palaeopathology was never very strong and he published little else on the subject. His last papers on the subject, in 1895, were on the pathology in Pleistocene mammals and on some pathology in the femur of Pithecanthropus. (Über einen Besuch der West-fällischen Knochenhöhle, *Zeitschrift für Ethnologie, Berlin*, 1870, 22, 365 (footnote); Untersuchung des Neanderthal Schädels, *ibid*, 1872, 4, 57; Knochen vom Höhlenbären mit krankhaften Veränderungen, *ibid*, 1895, 17, 706–8; Exostosen under Hyperostosen von extremitäten-knochen des Meuschen im Hinblick auf den Pithecanthropus, *ibid*, 1895, 17, 787–93.

5. F. Ivanhoe, Was Virchow right about Neanderthal? *Nature*, 1970, 227, 577–9.

6. S. Jarcho, The development and present condition of human palaeopathology in the United States, In: *Human palaeopathology*, edited by S. Jarcho, New Haven, Yale University Press, 1966, p 5. Even as late as 1968, the skeletal report on the skeletons from the Romano-British cemetery at Trentholme Drive in York contained eight pages of tables derived from cranial measurements. (R. Warwick, Bone pathology and abnormality, In: *The Romano-British cemetery at Trentholme Drive, York*, London, HMSO, 1968, pp 158–71.

7. Warren's first observations were published as an appendix to his *Comparative view of the sensorial and nervous systems in man and animals*, Boston, Ingraham, 1822. The appendix was entitled *Account of the crania of some of the aborigines of the United States*, pp 129–44. Morton published his findings in *Crania Americana*, Boston, Dobson; and Jones his in *Explanations of the aboriginal remains in Tennessee*, Washington, Smithsonian Institution, 1876.

8. Jarcho, *op cit*, pp 1–15.

9. Moodie, *op cit*; L. Pales, *Palèopathologie et pathologie comparative*, Masson, Paris, 1930; M.A. Ruffer, *Studies in the palaeopathology of Egypt*, Chicago, University of Chicago Press, 1921. Ruffer's book was the first volume to be given over entirely to palaeopathology.

10. Moodie also contributed a biographical sketch and a bibliography of Ruffer to the book, and this remains the most comprehensive account of the life and work of this most important figure in the history of palaeopathology. Sandison wrote an appreciation to Ruffer to mark

the 50th anniversary of his death but the definitive biography is still awaited. (A.T. Sandison, Sir Marc Armand Ruffer (1859–1917). Pioneer of palaeopathology, *Medical History*, 1967, 11, 150–6.)

11. M.A. Ruffer, On pathological lesions found in Coptic bodies (400–500 AD), *Journal of Pathology and Bacteriology*, 1913, 18, 149–62.

12. Moodie, *op cit*, p 21.

13. R.W. Schufeldt, Notes on palaeopathology, *Popular Science Monthly*, 1893, 42, 679–84.

14. E.A. Hooton, *The Indians of Pecos Pueblo: a study of their skeletal remains*, New Haven, Yale University Press, 1930.

15. The origin of syphilis still looms large in palaeopathology, especially whether it truly was a New World import into Europe. The evidence for this view is presented by B.J. Baker and G.J. Armelagos, The origin and antiquity of syphilis, *Current Anthropology*, 1988, 29, 703–20. Recently, skeletons of pre-Columbian date with syphilis have been reported in Europe. See, for example, A. Stirland, Pre-Columbian treponematosis in medieval Britain, *International Journal of Osteoarchaeology*, 1991, 1, 39–47.

16. Pales, *op cit*, p 6. Angel's phases differ somewhat from those of Pales. He included everything up to the turn of the century as a first phase ushering in a second, creative, phase which ended with the First World War. In Angel's scheme there followed a period of depression which was reversed by Hooton. (J.L. Angel, History and development of paleopathology, *American Journal of Physical Anthropology*, 1981, 56, 509–15.)

17. J.G. Roney, Palaeopathology of a California archaeological site, *Bulletin of the History of Medicine*, 1959, 33, 97–109.

18. Hooton, *op cit*, p 307, table X-1.

19. Amongst those whom Roney picked out for special mention were Krogman, Angel, Goldstein, Vallois and Todd; the references to the specific papers are to be found in Roney's 1959 paper, *op cit*, pp 108–9.

20. Roney's main conclusions are contained in the 1959 paper but they were also published in an abbreviated form in 1966 with an interesting discussion by A.M. Bunes, S.F. Cook and J.E. Anderson. (J.G. Roney, Palaeoepidemiology: an example from California, In: *Human palaeopathology*, edited by S. Jarcho, New Haven, Yale University Press, 1966, pp 99–107, discussion pp 107–20.)

21. H.U. Williams, The origin of syphilis: evidence from diseased bones, *Archives of Dermatology and Syphilis*, 1936, 33, 783–7. In fact the decline may have begun even sooner for Hooton himself noted (*op cit*, p 305), 'The pathology of dry bones is a sadly neglected field of investigation. The clinicians of to-day manifest but slight interest in the subject'.

22. Jarcho, *op cit*, p 24.

23. Angel, *op cit*, p 511. The transcript of Jarcho's symposium was published the following year (Jarcho, *op cit*), Brothwell and Sandison, *op cit*. The Paleopathology Association was founded after the unwrapping and autopsy of the mummy PUM II in Detroit (A. Cockburn, R.A. Barrato, T.A. Reyman and W.H. Peck, Autopsy of an Egyptian mummy, *Science*, 1975, 187, 1115–60). Cockburn was an epidemiologist who is now best remembered for his book on the evolution of the infectious diseases (*Infectious diseases: their evolution and eradication*, Springfield, C.C. Thomas, 1967) and the one co-authored with his wife, Eve, on mummies, for which he received a posthumous award from the American Writers Association (*Mummies, disease, and ancient cultures*, Cambridge, Cambridge University Press, 1980). For more details see J.L. Angel and M. Zimmerman, T. Aidan Cockburn, 1912–1981: A memorial, *American Journal of Physical Anthropology*, 1982, 58, 121–2.

24. Calvin Wells (1908–1978) was the most colourful practitioner of palaeopathology in the UK. His *Bones, bodies and disease* (London, Thames and Hudson, 1964) was the introduction to palaeopathology for many of those who later became more deeply involved and he was immensely kind to those at the start of their career, although he much preferred them to have a medical qualification. He was also probably the worst driver in the world and those who took the route from his cottage to the Castle Museum in Norwich must have felt that their time had come: I certainly did!

25. Peter Medawar spoke out strongly in favour of the use of imagination in science, and of the use of deduction rather than induction; see, for example, *Plato's republic*, London, Oxford University Press, 1984, pp 73–135.

26. I. Berlin, *Personal impressions*, edited by H. Hardy, Oxford, Oxford University Press, 1982, p 146.

27. O. Temkin, Palaeopathology and the history of medicine, In: *Human palaeopathology*, edited by S. Jarcho, New Haven, Yale University Press, 1966, pp 30–5.

28. A.C. Klebs, Palaeopathology, *Johns Hopkins Medical Bulletin*, 1917, 1, 2261–6.

29. E.R. Kerley and W.M. Bass, Paleopathology: meeting ground of many disciplines, *Science*, 1967, 157, 638–44.

2
The Nature of the Sample

Epidemiology is the study of disease in a community. In a modern context, action may sometimes be taken on the basis of the findings of an epidemiological investigation—an intervention of some kind, or the introduction of a new form of treatment for a particular disease—and thus a major part of any epidemiological investigation is taken up with ensuring that the population being studied is representative of the larger group from which it is taken in order to avoid bias which may precipitate a course of action which may not be truly justified: the banning of a useful medicine, for example. Bias is the bane of the modern epidemiologist; errors are acceptable since one can usually rely on the statisticians to supply the necessary corrective measures; but bias, that is a systematic error which disturbs the outcome of the study, is difficult to control and sometimes may not even be noticed at all.

Palaeoepidemiologists do not need to suffer from any anxieties that their work may have unfortunate, perhaps even dangerous, consequences since the worst they can do is to cause some misleading information to appear in the journals which accept their work; they are not likely adversely to affect public health policy, or alter prescribing habits or lead to the banning of potentially dangerous work practices. They do owe it to themselves and their potential editors and readers to consider sources of bias, however, or at least be aware of them in their work and plan and interpret their investigations accordingly.

In modern practice, samples for epidemiological study are typically drawn at random from a much larger population unless the population itself is sufficiently small that all its members can be studied. This might be the case in a cross-sectional study of a group of workers in a factory, for example, although this engenders a further question, that is, to what extent is this group—of painters, say—representative of painters as a whole? This question need not be pursued here; those who are anxious to know how to deal with it should consult a standard text.[1]

The methods employed in drawing a sample from a population[2] vary but there is invariably some attempt to use random methods in the selection so that, in theory, each member of the population has an equal chance of being selected so long as no other constraints apply; and they frequently do, the principal being the time which is allotted to the study and the amount of money available to fund it. Thus in a population with a skewed age and sex distribution it would be important to ensure that this was reflected in the sample so that the conclusions drawn about the sample would be true also of the population.

If the sample is selected properly the chance of bias, that is, of *systematic* error, operating will be greatly reduced, although probably not entirely eliminated, and the results will be that much more reliable.

The population which may be used in palaeoepidemiology will almost never be random in any sense to which an epidemiologist would willingly subscribe, although it is perfectly possible to derive a random sample from it; no one should be deceived into thinking that this does anything to offset any bias inherent in the parent sample, however, or that the results of the study are somehow purified by the process.

Bias is almost inevitable in palaeoepidemiological populations (meaning, here, the skeletons actually available for study) for a variety of reasons, the most obvious of which is that we have no control over their selection because of a number of what one might call extrinsic and intrinsic factors to which we must now give some attention.

EXTRINSIC FACTORS

The aim of a palaeoepidemiology study is to be able to make some general statements about a whole population based on the observations made on a sample that was once part of this whole. The whole population comprises all those who died in the location at a certain time; it is another question as to how far this dead population reflects reality in the corresponding living population and we shall return to that later.

There are four extrinsic factors which act on the dead population and they are extrinsic in the sense that they are independent of any of the biological features of the population. They all tend to reduce the size of the sample so that the final number of individuals (or skeletons) available for study is smaller, and most likely very much smaller, than the original.

The four factors are (i) the proportion of those dying who are buried at the site being studied, (ii) the proportion of those buried who survive to discovery, (iii) the proportion discovered and (iv) the total recovered. The five sub-groups involved are shown diagrammatically in Figure 2.1.[3] The magnitude of the proportions lost at each stage (p1–p4) will vary one from the other in a manner which will certainly not be constant and may not be known, although there is a better chance of estimating some than others, as we shall see.

The Proportion of Dead Buried at the Site

There is little that is random about the place in which one is buried, this being determined by place of domicile, religious beliefs and social mores amongst others; many will actually have chosen their burial place in advance. A burial assemblage, therefore, is a social or cultural sample, not a biological one, and to that extent may not in any way be typical of the population of which it was once a part.[4]

The proportion of the total dead population buried at a single spot will thus be at the whim of many and different influences, and estimates of this proportion are likely to be based on guesswork rather than anything more certain. There are exceptions of course:

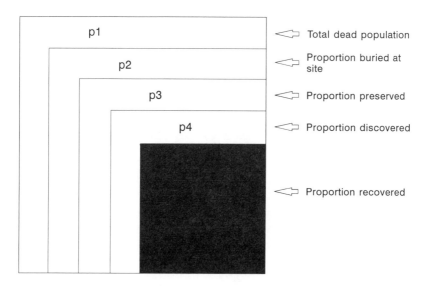

Figure 2.1 Model to show losses in skeletal numbers which occur at different stages. p1=proportion of total dead population in a buried population; p2=proportion of buried skeletons which are preserved; p3=proportion of skeletons discovered by the archaeologist; p4=proportion of those discovered which are actually recovered for examination

at some sites the number buried may include all those who died, at a battle or in a shipwreck or following some catastrophe, for example, but these will be exceptional cases. Where parish records exist for the site, especially if the parish is small and served by only one or two churches, and if phasing of the site is sufficiently tight, an estimate of the proportion may be possible, although allowance will have to be made for the loss due to disturbance and poor preservation.

Proportion Lost due to Disturbance and Poor Preservation

Bodies buried in a cemetery are rarely left undisturbed for long; this is especially the case in towns where the press of people and their insatiable demand for space results in an intense pressure on the accommodation provided for their predecessors. There is plentiful historical evidence for this and it can readily be confirmed by studying the site plans of any cemetery dig where grave-cuts are obvious even to the most cursory examination.[5]

The fully preserved, gleaming white skeleton is a thing which survives only in the minds of writers of fiction; the reality is quite likely to be something which resembles well chewed digestive biscuit and which may be about as easy to deal with.

The factors which govern decomposition and skeletonisation and the subsequent preservation of the skeleton have been thoroughly studied, especially by forensic scientists to whom these matters are of especial interest.[6] Decomposition of the body does appear to be amenable to some reasonably constant explanations, being aided by dry, aerobic conditions, for example; in optimum circumstances, a body may be skeletonised in four to six months and only then do problems arise for those wishing to study the bones.

Taphonomy, that is, the events leading to the disruption and loss of skeletal elements, has been most thoroughly studied by animal bone specialists who have generally confirmed the classic study of Brain who showed that small bones are likely to disappear from an animal carcase together with the cartilaginous ends of long bones, and that hard, dense bone survives well, often because it defeats the efforts of dogs to chew it.[7]

The taphonomy of human bone has not been studied with anything like the same enthusiasm but a study of a Romano-British cemetery in London showed that the survival of different bones was highly variable—as one would expect. Dense bones like the petrous temporal, the mandible and the heads of the humerus and femur survived well; anterior bones like the pubis and sternum survived poorly; and the small bones of the hands and feet were also likely to be markedly under-represented.[8] These findings are consistent with those of Brain and subsequent workers and have also been largely corroborated by the more recent study of human bones by Mays.[9]

The net result of the processes of taphonomy and human activity in the graveyard is that many skeletons are found in a somewhat bedraggled state with elements missing, and this may have unfortunate consequences when an attempt is made to decide which diseases are present. In still other cases, the burial is represented merely by a coffin stain, all of what Todd optimistically called 'the indissoluble bone'[10] having dissolved to nothing.

The Proportion Discovered

Where they are not obliterated by them, burial grounds are often obscured by modern civil engineers and, it must be said, by less modern ones. The archaeologist is only able to recover those burials that are within the power of his trowel to uncover and this proportion is subject to considerable variation and may not be constant through time, even at one site. Figure 2.2 shows a simple model to illustrate this. Here, there is a hypothetical site with three well-defined phases with an equal number of burials in each phase, but the proportion of burials discovered in each is different and, in this example, actually increases as one proceeds forward through the phases. In reality the proportion discovered may vary in any direction at any time and be completely unknown. What is more likely to be known, however, from a survey of the site, or

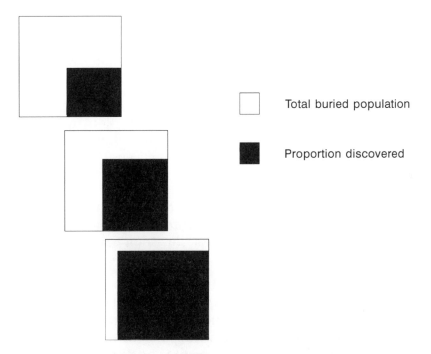

Total buried population

Proportion discovered

Figure 2.2 Model to show varying proportions of buried population which are discovered. In the model, the total numbers in the three cases are the same but the proportions discovered vary greatly. There is usually no way of knowing what proportion the discovered number is of the total

from trial excavations or from documentary sources, is the total extent of the cemetery and the proportion which has been excavated. It may thus be possible to make some kind of estimate of the likely maximum occupancy of the cemetery which may not be much more than a single order of magnitude in error.

Proportion Excavated

This step should involve the least loss and ought to be the single one which can be quantified reasonably accurately. There are always some skeletons which are too fragile to excavate but at worst a site diagram or a photograph can be studied and sex and obvious pathology may be evident. At best, the bone specialist (or some other competent person) will be on site to examine the skeleton *in situ* and not everything will be lost. There is a potential for further attenuation of numbers during washing, packing and despatch but these losses should be few and discernible and ought not to complicate an already perfectly awful situation much further.

INTRINSIC FACTORS

The only intrinsic factor which needs to be considered in the present context is that we are dealing of necessity with a dead rather than a living population; this may seem so blindingly obvious that it does not need saying but it is surprising how often this fact is overlooked.

Dead populations differ in some important respects from living ones, particularly in respect of their age structure. Moreover, they differ according to stage of economic development.

Figure 2.3 shows the demographic profile of some contemporary living populations from countries in varying stages of development. In each case there is a high proportion of young people in the population but the proportion in the older age groups increases with increasing development (in the figure, from Peru to England and Wales). The age distribution of a dead population (Figure 2.4) in a developing country is typically U-shaped with a lot of deaths occurring at both extremes of the age range. The effect of an improving economy is to reduce the number of deaths which

(a) Peru

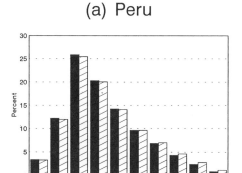

(b) Sri Lanka

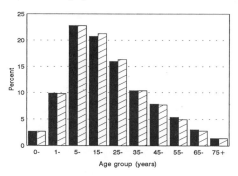

(c) England & Wales

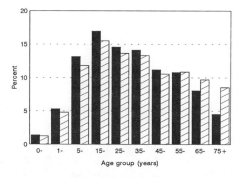

Figure 2.3 Percentage age distribution of living populations from (a) Peru, (b) Sri Lanka and (c) England and Wales in 1989 for males (black bars) and females (shaded bars). These are taken as examples of an undeveloped, a developing and a developed country, respectively. It will be noted that the proportion of young people in the population decreases and that of the elderly increases as a country becomes more developed

(a) Peru

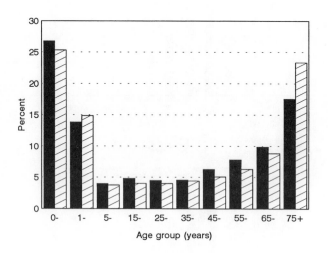

(b) Brazil

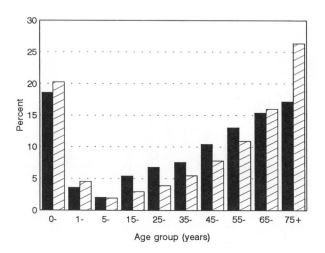

(c) Sri Lanka

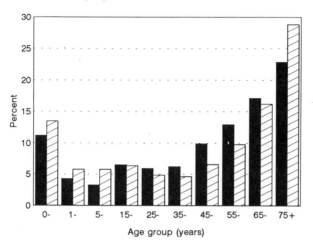

(d) England & Wales

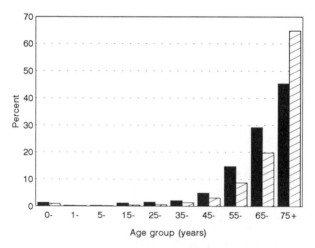

Figure 2.4 Percentage age distribution of total number of deaths occurring in (a) Peru, (b) Brazil, (c) Sri Lanka and (d) England and Wales in 1989 for males (black bars) and females (shaded bars). In an undeveloped country (Peru) the age distribution is U-shaped with many deaths occurring at both extremes of age. As the countries become increasingly developed (Brazil and Sri Lanka) the number of deaths in infancy and childhood progressively decreases and in a fully developed country (England and Wales) the distribution is skewed heavily to the right and there are very few deaths (relatively) below the age of 45 years. (Note that Brazil does not appear in Figure 2.3 since data were not available for the living population when these figures were being prepared)

occur amongst the young so that eventually the distribution is skewed markedly to the right, as seen for England and Wales in the figure. The most typical U-shaped curve is shown for Peru, with Brazil and Sri Lanka occupying intermediate positions between these two.

Palaeopathological populations will not be exactly comparable to any modern society but we might expect that their demographic features will be much more like those of an under-developed or developing country and that the distribution of the population will approximate much closer to those than to that of contemporary England and Wales.[11]

It is necessary to remember when drawing inferences from the demography of a palaeopathological population that the comparison is with a dead and not a living population and that although it is, of course, related to the living population from which it was drawn, since the form of the relationship is not known it will not be possible to reconstruct the demography of the living population. In epidemiological terms, in palaeopathology one is dealing with a closed (static) population rather than an open (dynamic) one. This difference must be borne in mind when discussing the prevalence of diseases (as will be discussed in Chapter 4) and when drawing inferences from life tables.

Assigning an age to a mature skeleton is no easy task and although some accord ages to skeletons with a precision and a confidence which is at best reckless, most know that ten-year age bands are about as close as one is likely to get. It follows that any life tables constructed from a skeletal sample will suffer from a wide margin of error, although it can be shown that under ideal conditions life expectancies calculated for dead and living populations can agree closely.[12] Unless the investigator remembers the basis of his calculations, however, he may be drawn into making some nonsensical remarks. Thus one author, in commenting on features of a life table derived from a skeletal assemblage, says in describing the various columns in it that 'l(x) simply represents survivorship. Of the 100% initial population ... at age 0, only approximately 79.9% were alive for their first birthday, approximately 77.8% for their second, etc.'[13] The truth is that *none* of those represented in the table at age 0 survived to see one birthday, let alone two, and while one might excuse this solecism as a piece of short-hand, it does show that the true nature of the sample, the procedure being carried out and the conclusions drawn from it were not as clear as they ought to have been; and this is by no means an isolated case.

TIME SCALES

While discussing the differences between palaeopathological populations and those with which epidemiologists usually choose to work, it is just worth mentioning time scales. In epidemiological studies, time scales are generally reckoned in decades at most; a big follow-up study of a sample designed to measure the incidence of a disease might operate over thirty years (although the study would be carried out in substantially less time using techniques described in Chapter 4) but this is about the upper end of the range; most studies would operate over much shorter periods. The populations available to the palaeoepidemiologist, by contrast, may—and usually do—represent individuals who died many hundreds of years apart and although good phasing may be able to divide the group into sub-units which belong to shorter periods, a hundred or two years is about as short an interval as is likely to be achieved. There are some exceptions where the date of death can be much more precisely determined or in which the deaths are known to have taken place over a short time: plague pits, crypt burials and battle cemeteries are examples, but none of these is common.

This extended time scale with which one has, of necessity, to work has the effect of smoothing out differences within and between groups, as is illustrated in Figure 2.5. In this fictitious example, there were two episodes of markedly increased prevalence of a disease over a comparatively short time, which we might assume was due to the operation of some environmental factor; because the data are studied for the entire period, these two interesting features are obscured. The overall effect is to produce a mean prevalence rate for the period (11.2) which is higher than the population actually experienced over the entire period, with the exception of the two crisis periods. Were the position to be reversed,

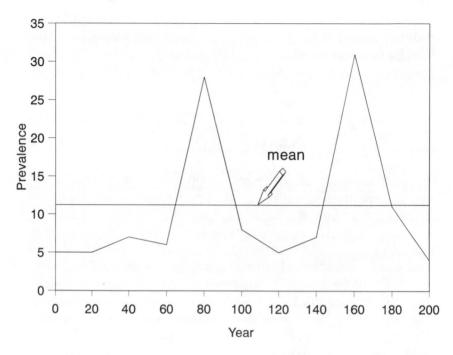

Figure 2.5 Hypothetical prevalence of a disease over time. There are two greatly increased peaks of prevalence which tend to elevate the mean prevalence above the usual rate. In a palaeopathological study, the peaks are likely to escape recognition and it will be impossible to correct for their influence on the mean. It will be noted that if there are trends of abnormally low prevalence, the observed prevalence may be lower than was usually the case

that is, had there been periods during which the prevalence rates were substantially lower than usual, the net effect would have been to *reduce* the mean. There is no *a priori* means of knowing whether the prevalence rate in a palaeopathological population is higher or lower than its 'real' value and so no way to correct the observed rate.

Thus we are dealing with a population: which has suffered and died from diseases that are largely non-random; which is a social or cultural and not a biological sample; which is an unknown proportion of the total dead population; and which has suffered a number of depredations in the time between burial and recovery. Most epidemiologists would at this stage be regretting ever leaving such simple matters as trying to trace cohorts of workers from factory records; the palaeoepidemiologist, however, has no choice but to proceed as he is not going to get anything better to work on. To be a bit more encouraging, there are some checks and balances which can be made.

For example, the age and sex structure of any skeletal population can be determined to see whether it fits to expectation; that is, is the distribution analogous to the knowledge of the stage of development at the time? Most pre-industrial societies are likely to have a distribution which is more or less U-shaped (see Figure 2.4), with a substantial number of juveniles, perhaps up to 30%. If this is not the case, then unless there are good reasons for this—the infants were buried elsewhere, as in the Romano-British period, for example—one should think hard before carrying out any extensive epidemiological studies on it.

Secondly, the sex ratio of the adults can be checked; this should not vary much from unity without a good explanation which is known beforehand. It is an interesting observation, for example, that Romano-British populations frequently have an excess of males, but the explanation for this is unclear (Table 2.1).[14]

Table 2.1   Sex ratios at some Romano-British cemeteries

Site	Per cent		Ratio M : F	N^a
	Male	Female		
Ilchester	63	27	2.3	43
Queensford Mill	40	60	0.7	57
Cassington	66	34	1.9	64
West Tenter Street	68	32	2.1	84
Victoria Road	61	39	1.6	85
Dunstable	53	47	1.1	86
Ashton	70	30	2.3	166
Lankhills	61	39	1.6	183
Trentholme Drive	80	20	4.0	266
Cirencester	69	31	2.2	293
Butt Road	57	43	1.3	299
The Querns	71	29	2.4	345
Poundbury	46	54	0.9	804

Data from several sources.
[a]Number of adult skeletons of identified sex.

Where the sex ratio is markedly different from expected, the first uncharitable thought might be that some mistake has been made, unless the epidemiologist has also performed the routine anthropology; but unless the assemblage can be re-examined it would be sensible to move onto more promising material.[15]

SAMPLE SIZES

A question which is frequently asked is: 'Is the sample large enough?' The answer can only be: 'Large enough for what?' Some samples will never be sufficiently large to provide an adequate demographic profile—ten bodies could provide no useful information on this point for example. A hundred might, though, and ten samples of ten from closely related sites might also do so. In this case, a plot of the data would quickly show whether the result was more or less in accord with *a priori* expectations, and common sense (a commodity not to be scorned in the interpretation of data) would dictate the weight to be given to the observations.

There is no magic number above which a sample becomes 'large enough' but it is possible to calculate the numbers needed in some circumstances. For example, suppose that it was desired to know how many adult skeletons should be measured to obtain a reasonable estimate of the population mean for some parameter, then one could use the formula:

$$n= (Z_\alpha \times s/d)^2$$

where n = number of cases required, Z_α = the probability that the estimate will include the population parameter, s = the standard deviation of the parameter and d = the tolerance within which the mean is to be estimated.

The probability is customarily taken at 95%, in which case Z_α = 1.96 (from t-tables); d is arrived at on the basis of an arbitrary decision; s, however, poses a problem unless it is known from other studies. If the parameter to be estimated were the mean height of the population, it is very likely that previous work would have produced results which could be used; let us suppose we know from other studies that the standard deviation (s) of this measure is 8.0 cm for medieval males. Further, let us suppose we wish the estimated mean to be ±5 cm of the population mean; n is then simply derived as follows:

$$n = (1.96 \times 8.0/5)^2 \approx 10$$

This is a surprisingly small number. If, however, we wish for greater precision the numbers required rapidly increase. Thus for $d = 2$, $n = 62$; for $d = 1$, $n = 246$; while for $d = 0.5$, $n = 983$.[16]

Sample size is also critical when trying to measure differences between groups as one might do, for example, in a case-control study, but again there is a formula to hand which will supply the answer provided that some key bits of information can be fed into it. We will leave further reference to this matter until Chapter 6, however, and proceed to the next area of difficulty, the question of diagnosis.

NOTES

1. For example, R.R. Monson, *Occupational epidemiology*, 2nd edition, Boca Raton, CRC, 1990.
2. The reader should be aware of the potential for confusion here since these terms can be used interchangeably, although in epidemiology they have more precise meanings. A population is usually taken to mean the entire group (often a mathematical abstraction) of those potentially available for study and a sample is some proportion of it chosen at random for the sake of expediency and of getting a study done in a manageable time. The sample is used to estimate population parameters. This issue is discussed further by D.W. Read, Archaeological theory and statistical methods: discordance, resolution, and new directions, In: *Quantitative research in archaeology. Progress and prospects*, edited by M.S. Aldenderfer, Newbury Park, Sage Publications, 1987, pp 151–84.
3. A similar scheme with respect to assemblages of animal bones has been discussed by T.J. Ringrose, Bone counts and statistics: a critique, *Journal of Archaeological Science*, 1993, 20, 121–57.
4. This point can be exemplified by considering a community with a mix of people of different national origins or religions. The individuals buried in the Methodist or Baptist or Jewish cemeteries might not be typical of the population as a whole; similarly, we can imagine that a buried population discovered in Tower Hamlets in years to come which was derived from the Bangladeshi immigrants would

give an impression of the population of the London borough, which was certainly skewed in some parameters.

5. Further details are to be found in C. Gittings, *Death, burial and the individual in early modern England*, London, Routledge, 1984, especially Chapter 5. Ruth Richardson quotes the *Commons Journal* for 1746–7 as saying of two London churchyards that they 'are so full of Corps, that it is difficult to dig a Grave without digging up some parts of a Corps before decayed...' (*Death, dissection and the destitute*, London, Penguin Group, 1988, p 79).

6. A.K. Mant has been one of the foremost investigators in this area and his principal research formed the basis of his University of London MD Thesis, *A study in exhumation*, 1950. A more accessible summary is to be found in Knowledge acquired from post-war exhumations. In: *Death, decay and reconstruction* (in: A. Boddington et al, *op cit*), pp 65–78.

7. C.K. Brain, *The hunters or the hunted? An introduction to African cave taphonomy*, Chicago, University of Chicago Press, 1981, pp 11–29.

8. T. Waldron, The relative survival of the human skeleton: implications for palaeopathology. In: A. Boddington, A.N. Garland and R.C. Janaway (editors), *Approaches to archaeology and forensic science*, Manchester, Manchester University Press, 1987 pp 55–64.

9. S. Mays, Taphonomy (*sic*) factors in a human skeletal assemblage, *Circaea*, 1992, 9, 54–8.

10. T.W. Todd, Skeletal records of mortality, *Scientific Monthly*, 1927, 24, p 482.

11. Historians have also studied this issue and many see parallels between the populations of medieval and post-medieval cities and cities in the developing world. See, for example, V. Perl, Change and stability in seventeenth-century London, In: *The Tudor and Stuart town*, edited by J. Ray, London, Longman, 1990, pp 139–65.

12. The life expectancy based on the data published by OPCS for the total living population of England and Wales and on all deaths in the same year is virtually identical. For example, using the data for 1984, the life expectancy of males at birth, calculated from the live population, was 73.3 whereas that calculated from all deaths was 70.9.

13. A. Boddington, From bones to populations: the problem of numbers. In: A. Boddington et al, *op cit*, p 182.

14. At Cirencester, Calvin Wells suggested that the large excess of males which was found (approximately 2:1) was because the town was 'largely given over to retired legionaries ... many of whom lacked regular wives and whose sexual partners, if any, were probably drawn from the professional prostitutes who were no doubt an abundant and pleasant amenity of the town'. Regrettably, none of this delightful speculation can be verified. (The human burials, In:

Romano-British cemeteries at Cirencester, edited by A. McWhirr, L. Viner and Calvin Wells, Cirencester, Cirencester Excavation Committee, 1982, p 135.)

15. It must be recognised that some material may be so important that the epidemiological or statistical niceties will be of secondary (or even of no) consideration. There are very few archaeologists who would discount an assemblage of mesolithic skeletons on numerical grounds and palaeontologists are used to seeing ones or twos as quite large samples, even to the point of defining new species from such numbers. There is often a curious inverse relationship between the number in the sample and the number of investigators. The excavations of 28 American soldiers at Fort Erie in Canada, for example, was worked on by a team of 19 (*Snake Hill, an investigation of a military cemetery from the war of 1812*, edited by S. Pfeiffer and R.F. Williamson, Hamilton, Durn Press, 1991) whilst the ice-man may well set an all time record if the political wranglings surrounding his ownership can be settled (P.G. Bahn and K. Everett, Iceman in the cold light of day, *Nature*, 1993, 362, 11–12).

16. Further discussion on numbers can be found in S. Shennan, *Quantifying archaeology*, Edinburgh, Edinburgh University Press, 1988, Chapter 14.

3
The Question of Diagnosis

This book is about ways of measuring the frequency of disease in early populations using the evidence found in their skeletons. Before this can be done, however, there must be ways of recognising the diseases which are present and giving them a name which will enable others to recognise them also; in other words, they will need to be classified in some useful way. This classification is usually referred to as a diagnosis and it is with diagnosis that this chapter is concerned.

THE PURPOSE OF DIAGNOSIS IN CLINICAL PRACTICE

Diagnosis is one of the three bases of medical practice, the two others being prognosis and treatment. The purpose of diagnosis has always been to allow the physician to give a prognosis to his patient and suggest treatment. So far as we can tell, the manner of arriving at a diagnosis has changed very little in the course of medical history. First the physician would elicit the signs and symptoms presented to him by the patient and he might supplement these with some direct observations, either of the patient or of one his bodily fluids, most usually, until comparatively recently, the urine. Having got together as much information as he could, the physician would construct a differential diagnosis in which all the conditions which might conceivably give rise to some or all the signs and symptoms were mentally or actually tabulated. The intellectual task which then followed was to arrange the differential diagnoses in an order of probability and so arrive at the disease which was the most likely to be that from which his patient was suffering. Having made his decision the physician would inform the patient of the likely outcome and the extent to which this might be affected by treatment. The importance of the physician arriving at the correct diagnosis does not need emphasising since it could make the difference between treatment or not, perhaps between life and death. The antiquity of this procedure is attested to by the Edwin Smith papyrus which is thought to have been written around 1600 BC.[1] In this document the physician is instructed how to make the diagnosis, which is to be relayed to the patient with one of three verdicts: the illness would be

An ailment which I will treat;

An ailment with which I will contend; or

An ailment not to be treated.

Nothing much has changed in the intervening four or five thousand years except that the patient is now always examined, investigations have become vastly more complex and there have been important changes in treatment; whereas about forty years ago remedies were ineffective but harmless, they have now become effective but potentially very harmful.

On occasion the physician is not satisfied with a primary diagnosis and, instead, may seek a secondary one. For example, the diagnosis of gout depends upon demonstrating a number of signs and symptoms but especially a raised blood uric acid concentration. This may be due to an inborn inability to metabolise uric acid (so-called primary gout) but it may be due to a number of secondary causes. The diagnosis of gout, therefore, may not be sufficient in itself to allow treatment to begin; this may have to wait for the secondary diagnosis to be made. There are many other instances in which this would be the case.

THE NATURE OF DIAGNOSIS

The basis of diagnosis has always been rooted in the contemporary thinking about the aetiology of disease, the development of which can be roughly paraphrased as passing from what Sigerist has called the magico-religious[2] (spirits, demons and the little arrows of the Anglo-Saxons), through the humoral doctrine of the medieval period, the anatomico-pathological concepts of the late 18th and early 19th centuries, the infectious theories of the late 19th and early 20th centuries to the immunological notions of our own day.

To the lay mind, diagnosis has the air of a precise—if not an exact—science, but hardly anything could be further from the truth. The vocabulary of diagnosis is actually rather confused and imprecise and incorporates many different features or attributes of the patient's condition. Thus the diagnosis may simply be a symptom (biliary colic), a sign (jaundice), a description of a pathological organ (mitral stenosis), a clinical measurement (hypertension), an abnormal radiological appearance (osteopetrosis) or an abnormal laboratory result (hyperlipidaemia). In fact, the way in which diseases are classified reflects the uncertainty about what it is that really constitutes a disease in the first place and this accounts for the great variety of descriptions applied to it. Kendall has elegantly summed it up as

> rather like an old mansion which has been refurbished many times, but always without clearing out the old furniture first, so that amongst the new inflatable plastic settees and glass coffee tables are still scattered a few old Tudor stools, Jacobean dressers and Regency commodes, and a great deal of Victoriana.[3]

As Scadding has suggested, it is probably this lack of logical cohesion in our definition of individual diseases which has resulted in us being unable to produce a satisfactory definition of disease as a whole.[4]

To a very great extent this apparent confusion arises because, for the purposes of the practice of medicine, the name given to the disease does not much matter so long as it conveys what the doctor needs to know about the likely outcome and the direction his treatment should take. A diagnosis can be taken as a piece of medical short-hand for saying something like, 'this is the disease which will linger on and may get much worse unless I treat it with antibiotics'. We might call this disease lobar pneumonia but just as easily the lung disease treated with penicillin (or whatever is appropriate). The second description would lack a certain finesse, however, and might have to be modified somewhat to differentiate it from other lung diseases which are treated with antibiotics.

CHANGING FASHIONS IN DIAGNOSIS

One of the difficulties which faces those who are interested in the history of medicine, and particularly those who wish to detect temporal trends in disease, is that it is hard to compare like with like. Descriptions of symptoms may be inadequate and, except in the last sixty or seventy years or so, are extremely unlikely to be supplemented with any of the information which is so necessary nowadays for making a diagnosis, especially the results of laboratory tests and X-rays. Moreover, the original author is very likely to assume that his reader understands perfectly well what he means by 'rachisagra'[5] and, on this account, will not bother to go into too much detail about it; for those who come upon his work several decades, or several centuries later, the meaning may be completely incomprehensible. There is also an irresistible tendency amongst doctors to engage in 'splitting', that is, to render what once appeared to be one disease into ever smaller parts. This can be well illustrated by a consideration of the joint diseases.

Amongst the very early medical writers no distinction was drawn between any of the diseases which affect the joints; osteoarthritis, gout, rheumatoid arthritis, rheumatic fever and the others were all thought to be part of a single entity. This state of affairs continued until the late 16th century when Guillaume de Baillou made the distinction between gout and rheumatic fever and the other forms of arthropathy. Baillou was also the first to use the word rheumatism in anything like its modern sense. The distinction between gout and the other forms of joint disease was made very explicitly by Sydenham writing in the middle of the 17th century and his description of the pain as being like a dog gnawing is one with which modern sufferers can feel much sympathy. Cullen's description of rheumatism in the 18th century was notable for dividing the symptoms into those which were acute and affected the joints and muscles, and those which were chronic, affecting only the joints. This distinction was also maintained by Scudamore who, in 1827, published the first systematic treatise on rheumatism in English. Rheumatoid arthritis had probably been recognised as different from other forms of arthropathy during the 17th and 18th centuries but priority for differentiating it completely is generally given to Landrè-Beauvais who worked at the Salpêtrière in Paris and who gave the disease the name of *goutte asthénique primitive*. The concept of infectious arthritis was first suggested by Bouchard who noted that the joints were involved in many infectious diseases; he coined the term *pseudorheumatismes infectieux* for them and divided them into those in which the organism was known and those in which it was not. It is interesting to note here, however, that the arthropathy associated with gonorrhoea had been known of since the 16th century when swelling of the knee joint in association with urethritis and orchitis was noted by Petrus Forest of Alkmaar. This association was also well recognised during the 18th century, which was something of a golden age for the venereal diseases. Descriptions of ankylosing spondylitis appear during the 19th century but not until the later years of that century were accurate clinical descriptions first published, particularly by Marie and by Strümpell. It was not until 1904, however, that it was clearly distinguished from other spondylarthropathies.

The first complete clinical account of osteoarthritis was given by Cruveilhier in 1829 although illustrations of bones affected by the disease are to be found in the works of earlier authors, notably those of Sandiforts of Leyden, Eduard and Gerard. The osteophytes seen around the joint were described as arising *ex morbo rheumatico*. Later accounts were published by Colles, Smith and Adams in Dublin, and by Canton in England who gave an excellent account of osteoarthritis of the shoulder joint, calling it chronic rheumatic arthritis. Further accounts were given in the latter part of the 19th century by Deville, Broca and Weber, and by Virchow who is generally considered to have been the first to use the term *arthritis deformans* for this condition.[6]

So by the beginning of the 20th century, a number of separate conditions were known to affect the joints, some of which were subdivided into acute and chronic forms. Acute rheumatism was generally taken to mean only rheumatic fever while amongst the chronic forms were osteoarthritis, gout, rheumatoid arthritis and some forms of infectious arthropathy.

The most significant trend in recent times has been the recognition of the sero-negative arthropathies. Before the 1950s it was thought that rheumatoid arthritis was a non-specific syndrome which might be triggered off by a number of different aetiological factors such as psoriasis, urethritis or ulcerative colitis. During the 1950s these variants of classical rheumatoid arthritis came to be seen as discrete entities and this view was strengthened by the demonstration that serum from patients with these disorders did not contain an immunoglobulin which was found in patients with rheumatoid arthritis and which came to be known as rheumatoid factor; the condition in which rheumatoid factor was absent came to be known as the sero-negative arthropathies.

What I hope this brief survey has shown is that diagnosis is dependent upon aetiological concepts; before the discovery of micro-organisms the notion of infection as a cause of joint disease was impossible; similarly, before the development of immunology, the idea of a sero-negative arthropathy was unimaginable.

Changing fashions in diagnosis often make it extremely difficult to render diagnosis made in former times into their modern equivalents. This difficulty is compounded by the plethora of terms which may be used for the same condition. For example, osteoarthritis may be referred to in early writings as arthritis deformans, senile arthritis, morbus coxae senilis or as spondylitis deformans; nowadays the term osteoarthrosis is sometimes used as an alternative to osteoarthritis to escape the connotations of inflammation which the ending '-itis' implies, and some writers persist with the somewhat old-fashioned degenerative joint disease. Ankylosing spondylitis may also be found masquerading under the names of Marie-Strümpell disease, Bechterew's disease, bamboo spine, poker back, pelvospondylitis ossificans, rheumatismal ossifying pelvispondylitis, spondylarthritis ankylopoietica, atrophic ligamentous spondylitis, ossifying ligamentous spondylitis, rhizomelic spondylosis and, confusingly, spondylitis deformans. I dare not go on with any others, but you see the problem.

Those who read the early medical literature, therefore, must learn not to give diagnoses in these sources their modern meaning. Thus when Wood Jones writes in 1908 of the skeletons from Nubia that 'The disease which shows itself with by far the greatest frequency ... is rheumatoid arthritis'[7] we might express considerable surprise unless we realise that he is actually referring to what we would now call osteoarthritis; in which case we have no reason to disagree with him.[8]

It is not surprising that some modern palaeopathologists take the view that the only way to know what was meant by the descriptions in the old literature is to re-examine the bones, if indeed they are still available for study.

MAKING A DIAGNOSIS

The clinician relies on three sources of information to make his diagnosis: the patient's history which amongst other things will tell him what symptoms the patient has; the clinical examination from which he will elicit a number of signs; and a range of supplementary examinations which will include laboratory tests, radiography and pathology. The diagnosis may sometimes be made on the basis of the patient's history alone or it may be made only after the most exhaustive series of supplementary examinations—and it is the patient who is usually most exhausted at the end of them. The clinician uses the information he obtains to follow a diagnostic algorithm, although he may be unaware that this is what he is actually doing since the steps through the sequence may be taken subconsciously and he is working always to find the most parsimonious explanation for the data which he has to hand. Classically, medical students are taught to construct a differential diagnosis, that is, a list of *all* the diseases which might conceivably account for the patient's condition. These are then structured in such a way that they come to be arranged in order of probability, the final being the most probable and—by inference—the one with which the patient is afflicted. In practice, this long-winded approach is frequently circumvented except during formal case presentations when it is incumbent upon the presenter to outdo the audience in finding the most rare conditions to include in the differential.

For some diseases criteria have been developed which must be satisfied before a diagnosis can be made. Those for the

Table   3.1   Criteria   for   classification   of
spondylarthropathies

1	Inflammatory spinal pain
2	Synovitis
3	Family history
4	Psoriasis
5	Inflammatory bowel disease
6	Alternating buttock pain
7	Enthesopathy
8	Acute diarrhoea
9	Urethritis
10	Sacroiliitis

Based on Dougados *et al.*[9]

spondylarthropathies are shown in Table 3.1.[9] Of the ten criteria listed in the table, only two, enthesopathy and sacroiliitis, are at all amenable to demonstration in skeletal material. And this, of course, is the problem when attempting to make a diagnosis based on clinical criteria on skeletal material; there is simply too little information: no signs, no symptoms, no soft tissues to examine (except in the case of mummified bodies and these are the exception rather than the rule) and a rather limited set of supplementary examinations. And when it is remembered that in an average rheumatology clinic perhaps a quarter of the patients may never receive a final diagnosis at all, some doubts must be raised about the wisdom of trying it all on dry bones. On the bright side, there are some advantages which the palaeopathologist has over his clinical colleagues, and these will be mentioned later on.

THE ACCURACY OF DIAGNOSIS

Those with no experience of diagnosing disease in the living often have an exaggerated idea of its capabilities; there is a view that diagnostic compartments are completely separate entities and that every constellation of signs and symptoms fits neatly into one, and only one, box. The boundaries between diseases (even between health and disease) are frequently blurred and may overlap; pathological processes are dynamic, advancing, relapsing, and the final nature of a disease may not be known until several weeks or months after it has first been declared in the patient. In a substantial proportion of all cases, a diagnosis is never made or a euphemism may be applied to appease the patients who gain some reassurance from the fact that their doctors appear to know what is ailing them, or to save the doctors the embarrassment of having to admit their failure.

Having made a diagnosis, what are the chances of it being accurate? Regretfully, they are not very high. Several studies have been made of the accuracy of clinical diagnosis and they confirm what everyone knew but was reluctant to admit. In a study of 1117 cases which I carried out some years ago, in less than half was the clinical diagnosis confirmed at autopsy. The remaining cases were split almost equally between those in which there was only a minor disagreement between the clinical diagnosis and the autopsy findings, and those in which the disagreement was total; the accuracy of diagnosis for some categories of disease is illustrated in Table 3.2.[10]

Table 3.2   Proportion of clinical diagnoses confirmed at autopsy

	Number diagnosed	Number confirmed	Percentage confirmed
Cardiovascular disease	459	250	54.4
Ischaemic heart disease	167	128	76.7
Cerebrovascular disease	87	33	37.9
Hypertension	38	19	50.0
Pulmonary embolus	28	3	10.7
Malignant disease	244	122	50.0
Bronchial carcinoma	48	37	77.1
Carcinoma of the bowel	16	6	37.5
Carcinoma of the breast	9	7	77.8

Data from Waldron and Vickerstaff.[10]

DIAGNOSIS IN PALAEOPATHOLOGY

In making a diagnosis in palaeopathology, reliance in the majority of cases can be given only to the gross appearances and to radiology; it is a sadly depleted list compared with the information in the hands of the clinicians, who even then are not very good at it. Moreover, many of the vital pieces of evidence available to the clinician are also usually lacking and the disease is, of course, entirely static, the appearances being as they were at a particular unfortunate moment for the individual, the time of his death.

There are a few pathognomonic lesions on bones, however, and it is now becoming possible to confirm some diagnoses by immunological methods, but the number of diseases to which these conditions apply is few.[11] Moreover, the radiological and clinical criteria used to diagnose joint disease (the category most commonly encountered by the palaeopathologist, if not always of the most interest) for therapeutic or epidemiological purposes have little application for palaeopathology.

The radiological diagnosis of osteoarthritis depends *inter alia* on demonstrating joint space narrowing, the presence of marginal osteophytes and sclerosis (corresponding to areas of eburnation in the bare bones). Juliet Rogers and her colleagues have shown that a poor correspondence exists between the radiological and palaeopathological diagnoses of osteoarthritis of the knee. A series of 24 knee joints from 14 skeletons was assessed radiologically and pathologically. Eight were agreed to be normal by both methods, but of the remaining 16 considered abnormal by the palaeopathologist, only two were thought to be so by the radiologist. The principal difference between the two was that osteophytes were much more likely to be seen by visual inspection than by radiography; large osteophytes and eburnation, particularly in the patellar groove of the femur and on the anteroposterior aspects of the tibio-femoral joint, were often invisible to the radiologist. In this study the prevalence of osteoarthritis was 4% radiologically and 21% or 67% palaeopathologically, depending on the criteria used. Even using the more conservative of these last two figures, there is more than a fivefold difference in prevalence which does not bode well for comparative work.[12]

OPERATIONAL CRITERIA

'Diagnosis is by far the greatest problem [in palaeopathology]' Brothwell commented ruefully in 1961[13] and little has changed in the thirty years since he wrote these words since it should be apparent by now that palaeopathologists are not very likely to be able to outshine their clinical colleagues in diagnostic acumen and their chances of being able to make fine distinctions between different clinical entities must be reckoned somewhat slim. In many cases the most that will be achieved will be a broad classification of lesions, and lumping rather than splitting should be the norm in palaeopathology.[14]

If the results of palaeoepidemiological studies cannot be directly compared they will have little value (except presumably to the investigator) and authors should always refer to the source of the criteria used to make their diagnoses or, where there are no other published sources, give the criteria which they have used, just to give other investigators a sporting chance.

The most satisfactory solution—since, as we have seen, there may be little help to be gained from clinical experience—is to follow a standard epidemiological procedure and use operational criteria for classifying disease in the skeleton, accepting that they will differ (often profoundly) from those used by clinicians.[15] The reasons for this approach are not only that clinical and radiological criteria may not be applicable to the palaeopathologist but also that the palaeopathologist is able to see changes in the skeleton which the clinician and radiologist cannot. For example, it is common for the palaeopathologist to see osteoarthritic changes on the odontoid peg, but this is a site at which the disease is almost unknown to the clinician because the patient does not complain of pain in that joint and the radiologist is usually not concerned to visualise the changes there. Thus the information available to the palaeopathologist is different from that of his clinical colleagues and any classificatory system must take this into account.

It is obviously a major undertaking to make operational definitions for all the diseases which the palaeopathologist may come across in his study of bones but if something of the sort is *not* attempted the subject is likely to sink into epidemiological chaos as the possibility of making between-study comparisons will become more and more remote. The undertaking is not made any the less awesome given that the definitions will have to be acceptable to most, if not all, of those working in the field; they will have to be used by them and any refinements and changes which come about as our knowledge increases will similarly have to meet with general approval. It is not something which is likely to come about overnight.

We have made an attempt to produce some guidance towards this end for some joint diseases and some bone infections;[16] in the case of osteoarthritis we have published an operational definition. Osteoarthritis would be classified in the skeleton in the presence of eburnation or, if eburnation were absent, if *two* of the following were present in a joint: marginal osteophyte, pitting on the joint surface, alteration in the normal joint contour or new bone on the joint surface. In practice, not much would be lost, and indeed there would be less ambiguity if the classification were to rely *solely* on the presence of eburnation.[17]

The operational definition of osteoarthritis is straightforward and it is conceivable that there would not be too many voices raised in objection.[18] Arriving at operational definitions for other diseases likely to be encountered in palaeopathology, however, is much more challenging and it is not my purpose to attempt to do so here; I wish to do no more than point out the need to elaborate and to agree them, and then to encourage their use so that the process of classifying disease in palaeopathology will become less like trying to navigate through a minefield with the aid of the sun and a Mickey Mouse watch.

NOTES

1. H.E. Sigerist, *A history of medicine*, New York, Oxford University Press, volume 1, 1951, p 306.
2. Sigerist, *op cit*, p 267.
3. R.E. Kendall, *The role of diagnosis in psychiatry*, Oxford, Blackwell, 1975, p 20. Kendall also discusses the concept of disease and gives other references to this difficult area.
4. J.G. Scadding, Meaning of diagnosis in broncho-pulmonary disease, *British Medical Journal*, 1963, 2, 1425–30; The semantics of medical diagnosis, *Biomedical Computing*, 1972, 3, 83–90.
5. For those who do *not* know, it is an archaic word for backache.
6. There is no really comprehensive history of the joint diseases and I have leaned heavily on R.A. Stockman's account written in 1920 (*Rheumatism and arthritis*, Edinburgh, W. Green) for much of the

information in this section. His book contains some of the references to the original texts and others may be found in the list provided by W.S.C. Copeman in the introductory chapter to his *Textbook of the rheumatic diseases* (Edinburgh, Livingstone). The first edition of Copeman's book was published in 1948 and he edited the succeeding three editions (1955, 1964, 1969); J.T. Scott took over the editorship in 1978 for the 5th edition. It is extremely interesting to compare the chapters throughout the various editions to see how the concepts changed over time.

7. F. Wood Jones, Pathological report, In: *The archaeological survey of Nubia, Bulletin No 2*, Cairo, Ministry of Finance, 1908, p 55.

8. Some of the cases referred to as spondylitis deformans in the past were probably ankylosing spondylitis rather than osteoarthritis. This can sometimes be verified from photographs but otherwise this has to remain yet another area of uncertainty.

9. These are taken from M. Dougados, S. van der Linden, R. Juhlin, B. Huitfeldt, B. Amor, A. Calin, A. Cats, B. Dijkmans, I. Olivieri, G. Pasero, E. Verys and H. Zeidler, The European spondylarthropathy study group preliminary criteria for the classification of spondylarthropathy, *Arthritis and Rheumatism*, 1991, 34, 1218–27.

10. H.A. Waldron and L. Vickerstaff, *Intimations of quality. Ante-mortem and post-mortem diagnosis*, London, Nuffield Provincial Hospitals Trust, 1977.

11. Spondylolysis is one of the diseases which cannot be wrongly diagnosed in palaeopathology and the changes in the facial skeleton and in the hands and the feet in leprosy would be considered pathognomonic in their full-blown expression. Immunological techniques have been used to diagnose multiple myeloma by demonstrating the presence of myeloma protein (C. Cattaneo, K. Gelsthorpe, P. Phillips, T. Waldron, J.R. Booth and R.J. Sokol, Immunological diagnosis of multiple myeloma in a medieval bone, *International Journal of Osteoarchaeology*, 1994, 4, 1–2) and to isolate *Mycobacterium tuberculosis* using polymerase chain reaction (M. Spigelman and E. Lemma, The use of polymerase chain reaction (PCR) to detect *Mycobacterium tuberculosis* in ancient skeletons, *International Journal of Osteoarchaeology*, 1993, 3, 137–43. Using these immunological techniques it is possible only to *confirm* a diagnosis; a negative result will not necessarily lead to the rejection of a diagnosis since one cannot detect false negative results.

12. J. Rogers, I. Watt and P. Dieppe, Comparison of visual and radiographic detection of bony changes at the knee joint, *British Medical Journal*, 1990, 300, 367–8.

13. D. Brothwell, The palaeopathology of early man: an essay on the problems of diagnosis and analysis, *Journal of the Royal Anthropological Institute*, 1961, 91, 318–44.

14. Lumping is the process whereby entities are grouped together to make broader categories. For example, psoriatic arthropathy, Reiter's disease and enteropathic arthropathy can all be lumped together under the rubric of the sero-negative disorders.

15. It should perhaps be noted here that it is not only the palaeoepidemiologist who may find the application of clinical criteria unsatisfactory. It is very often the case that the modern epidemiologist is likewise inconvenienced because it is not always possible to incorporate physical examinations and laboratory and radiological tests into epidemiological studies. For further discussion see J.N. Katz and M.H. Liang, Classification criteria revisited, *Arthritis and Rheumatism*, 1991, 34, 1228–30.

16. J. Rogers, T. Waldron, P. Dieppe and I. Watt, Arthropathies in palaeopathology: the basis of classification into most probable cause, *Journal of Archaeological Science*, 1987, 14, 179–93; J. Rogers and T. Waldron, Infections in palaeopathology: the basis of classification into most probable cause, *ibid*, 1989, 16, 611–25.

17. I have used the term 'classification' in relation to describing disease in bones purposely to differentiate it from diagnosis, which has clinical overtones which are inappropriate in a palaeopathological context. The procedure differs so much between palaeopathology and clinical medicine that it seems to me to be much more useful to refer to it by a separate name.

18. There would certainly by no dissention to the diagnosis of osteoarthritis when eburnation was present. The discussion would centre round the extent to which the condition should be diagnosed when it was *not* present. There are some who advocate making the diagnosis on the basis of relatively minor changes; see, for example, M. Schultz, Paläopathologische Diagnostik, In: *Anthropologie. Handbuch der vegleichenden Biologie des Menschen,* edited by R. Knussmann, Stuttgart, Gustav Fischer, 1988, pp 480–96.

4
Measures of Disease Frequency

We have arrived at Chapter 4 with a sample that is subject to much bias of one sort or another and with a diagnostic process which might perhaps be thought of as about as accurate as a pack of Tarot cards. However, if we are to make any attempts at all to understand disease in the past, we have nothing *better* to work with and palaeopathologists can take some consolation from the fact that historians are often little better provided with raw data and are not distracted from their task and if we are aware of the potential biases in our material we can make allowances in the inferences we draw from it.

Having decided to carry on, the most important task which now faces the palaeoepidemiologist is to calculate the frequency of disease in his sample and this chapter will discuss how this should be done.

INCIDENCE AND PREVALENCE

There are a number of measures of disease frequency but the most important are incidence and prevalence. Incidence describes the number of new events occurring in a population within a specific time, whereas prevalence is the proportion of the population with a specified condition at any one time.

Incidence

Incidence (*I*) is calculated as:

$$\text{Incidence} = \frac{\text{Number of new cases}}{\text{Total population at risk}}$$

Since incidence has a time base it is a true rate and is generally expressed per 10^3 or 10^5 of the population at risk.

The numerator in the incidence equation is obtained by counting the number of new cases which occur during the observation period, which will, to some extent, be based on the nature of the disease under study; for a common acute infection such as influenza the observation period may be a week; for a rare disease or for one which has a long period of induction (which would include many cancers), the observation period may have to extend over many years.

The denominator in the equation, the population at risk, will include only those individuals who do not already have the disease. To return to the influenza example again: if the incidence rate were being calculated for one week, then those who had already contracted it and were suffering on the day the observations began would be excluded from the denominator—neither would they be in the numerator.

Prevalence

The equation for calculating prevalence (*P*) has the form:

$$\text{Prevalence} = \frac{\text{Number of cases}}{\text{Total population}}$$

Prevalence is a simple proportion and is thus not a rate, although it is frequently referred to as such.

It will be seen that the denominators in the two equations are different, and in some cases may be substantially different, particularly when dealing with common diseases with a long duration.

Relationship between Incidence and Prevalence

The prevalence of a disease depends upon two factors, its incidence rate and its duration; the relationship approximates to:

$$P \approx I \times D$$

where D = the duration of the disease.

Where the duration is short, P and I may be very similar, as is the case in many of the common infectious diseases of childhood. Where the duration is long, P may be many times greater than I and this is the case in chronic diseases such as osteoarthritis.[1]

Epidemiological Methods for Measuring Incidence and Prevalence

Incidence

As has been said above, the determination of an incidence rate requires a period of observation, which may be short or long depending upon the natural history of the disease. The procedure involves defining a population to study, frequently referred to as a cohort, and then following it up carefully and counting the number of new cases of the disease in question. For example, the population may be all the school children in a London borough who are followed up for three months to determine how many get chicken pox, having excluded all those with the disease at the start of the study period.

This type of study is usually known as a prospective or cohort study, although the latter term has rather fallen out of favour now.

For acute infections this design is about as simple and straightforward as anything ever is in epidemiology. Consider, however, the investigator who wishes to study the induction of bladder cancer in men exposed to chemicals used in dye making. He will establish a study population which might be all men currently working in the appropriate industries and he will probably stipulate a minimum period of exposure, which might be six months or a year, to eliminate those with very trifling exposure. The only task now is to count the number of new cases of bladder cancer as they arise, but a colleague mentions that carcinoma of the bladder may take twenty to thirty years to develop. Since there are few investigators sufficiently altruistic to set up such a study for others to complete—and fewer grant-giving bodies willing to sponsor it—a way round this problem had to be devised. The trick in such an investigation is to define a historical cohort and follow it up over the necessary period, which also ends at some point in the past. In our dye workers example, the cohort may be established as all those working in the industry on, say, 1 January 1960 and the follow-up period might end on 31 December 1989, thirty years later. This type of study may be called a retrospective prospective study, or an historical cohort study.

Prevalence

Prevalence is measured using a cross-sectional method in which a population is defined and the number of individuals with the disease of interest is noted. If one were interested in the prevalence of back pain in office workers, the result would almost certainly differ depending when the study was carried out, as the number of persons with and without back pain might be expected to vary—if only slightly—from week to week, just as the number of fat globules in the salami depends upon where you slice it.

A distinction is sometimes made between point prevalence and period prevalence, depending on whether the time of observation is short or long, but this distinction has little relevance to palaeo-pathologists whose study period is invariably long.

Crude and age-specific measures

When calculated using the whole population as the denominator, the incidence or prevalence is known as the crude rate, but it may sometimes be of interest to calculate age-specific incidence or prevalence by breaking the population into age groups and using each as the denominator in turn. Age-specific rates are useful for comparative purposes, as will be discussed in the next chapter.

OTHER MEASURES OF MORBIDITY AND MORTALITY

There are several other measures of morbidity and mortality, some of which need briefly to be mentioned here, including proportional mortality and a number relating to events around childbirth.[2]

Proportional Mortality Ratio

The proportional mortality ratio (PMR) expresses the ratio of death from one or more causes to deaths from all causes. It is used in conventional epidemiology when there are difficulties with denominators. It is also possible to calculate proportional morbidity ratios, but this is done infrequently in modern epidemiology.

Adverse Events Associated with Childbirth

The most important adverse event associated with childbirth is death, either of the child or the mother, and several death rates are used depending when the death occurs. Although death strictly speaking is a state rather than a disease, it seems worthwhile describing these rates here because some are alluded to in the palaeopathological literature.

Those I will briefly describe are the maternal mortality rate, the stillbirth and perinatal mortality rates, and the neonatal and infant mortality rates.

Maternal mortality rate

This is the ratio of maternal deaths to the number of live births (living infants) in a year:

$$MMR = \frac{\text{Number of maternal deaths}}{\text{Number of live births}}$$

and is usually expressed per 10^4 or 10^5 live births per year.

The stillbirth rate

This is the proportion of fetal deaths to the number of live births and fetal deaths:

$$SBR = \frac{\text{Number of fetal deaths}}{\text{Number of live births} + \text{fetal deaths}}$$

expressed by 10^3 per year. This rate excludes miscarriages from the numerator, that is, losses occurring before the 28th week of gestation.

The perinatal mortality rate

This expresses the number of deaths occurring in the fetus after 28 weeks gestation plus deaths of infants in the first week of life as a proportion of all live births and fetal deaths of 28 weeks or more:

$$\text{PNMR} = \frac{\text{Number of fetal deaths} \geq 28 \text{ weeks} + \text{infant deaths} \geq 7 \text{ days}}{\text{Number of live births} + \text{fetal deaths} \geq 28 \text{ weeks}}$$

This is generally given per 10^3 and per year.

The infant mortality rate

This is the proportion of infants dying in the first year of life compared with all live births:

$$\text{IMR} = \frac{\text{Number of deaths during the first year}}{\text{Total number of live births}}$$

The neonatal mortality rate

This compares the number of deaths in the first 28 days of life with the number of live births:

$$\text{NNMR} = \frac{\text{Number of deaths} < 28 \text{ days}}{\text{Total number of live births}}$$

The IMR and the NNMR are conventionally given per 10^3 per year.

RATES FOR USE IN PALAEOPATHOLOGY

It should be obvious from what has been said so far that all palaeoepidemiological studies are cross-sectional in nature and therefore *cannot* be used to measure incidence, although this term is frequently used to describe disease frequency in skeletal populations. What is actually measured in any palaeoepidemiological study is prevalence and almost always period prevalence, the period frequently being a very long one.

Proportional morbidity rates (but not, of course, proportional mortality rates) can be used in palaeoepidemiology although it may not always be a simple matter to define morbidity since there is no sudden change from normal to abnormal appearances in bone; we are not dealing with a dichotomous variable but rather a sliding scale from 'normal' at one end to 'abnormal' at the other and the decision as to when the cross-over has taken place is often a matter of opinion rather than of fact. In any study of PMR, then, it would be incumbent on the investigators clearly to define their criteria of morbidity, especially if they were hoping that other workers might be able to confirm their observations.

Since all the rates relating to childbirth have a denominator which includes the number of live births, none is appropriate to palaeoepidemiology. The so-called stillbirth rates that are sometimes calculated in palaeoepidemiology, in which the number of fetal skeletons is related to the total number of children, is simply a prevalence in this case of the number of fetal skeletons amongst the totality of children. Rates which require numbers of *live* births in the denominator can never be calculated in palaeoepidemiology because there is no way to determine the number of individuals entering the population; this can only be done with a dynamic population in which there is potential for ingress—and egress—of individuals. The palaeoepidemiological population is—by contrast—a closed population in which the numbers are fixed and cannot change, except through the processes of attrition which were discussed in Chapter 2.[3]

PATTERNS OF AGE-SPECIFIC PREVALENCE RATES IN A POPULATION

The patterns of age-specific prevalence rates of a particular disease in a living population vary according to its incidence and duration and we need now to consider the patterns of some diseases and see to what extent they are reflected by prevalence rates in groups of skeletons. There are important differences between those diseases that do not contribute towards death and those that do, and so they will be dealt with separately.

Diseases that Do Not Contribute towards Death

Many of the diseases that fall into this class and which affect the skeleton are of long duration and the pattern that is seen in their age-specific prevalence rates depends upon the age groups in which they are incident. Broadly speaking these diseases are of two types, those in which new cases arise only—or predominantly—during childhood or adolescence (for example, spondylolysis, rickets and some of the skeletal dysplasias) and those in which new cases arise first during adult life and continue to do so at all subsequent ages; osteoarthritis is the prime example of this second type of disease.

We can take spondylolysis as the model for the first type. It arises in childhood and for the present purposes we can take it that cases do not arise thereafter.[4] The duration of the resulting lesion is for the lifetime of the individual; the prevalence rate thus increases from zero at (say) age 5 to a maximum at (say) age 20 and it remains at that rate for all subsequent ages (see Figure 4.1).[5] With increasing age some of those with the disease will die, thus decreasing the numerator, but the total numbers in the population will also be decreasing and hence the denominator will also reduce in size and the rate will, therefore, tend to remain relatively constant.

Taking osteoarthritis as the model for the second type of disease we see a completely different pattern. This disease tends to occur first in the late 20s or early 30s and the incidence increases steadily thereafter. Because the duration of the disease is for the lifetime of the individual, the prevalence increases markedly with age and in extreme old age there is almost no one who will not have at least one joint affected.

In cases where the disease does not (or does not materially) contribute towards death it is reasonable to suppose that the prevalence in a skeletal population is a reliable estimate of the prevalence in the living, as can be shown by a simple model. Consider any living population in which a proportion of the adults has osteoarthritis. Since this disease does not adversely affect survival to any significant degree, nor is it associated with any other condition which does, the fact of having osteoarthritis does not in itself contribute towards the probability of dying and so an individual with osteoarthritis is as likely or not to die as one without the disease. The proportion of those who die with osteoarthritis will thus be no different from the proportion of those

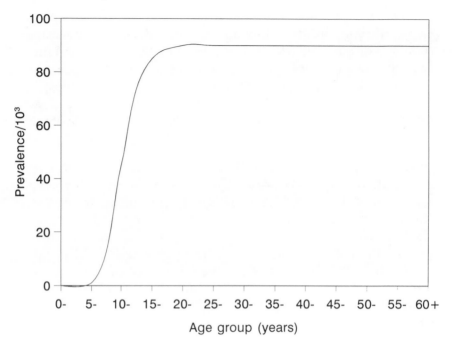

Figure 4.1 Hypothetical age-specific prevalence of spondylolysis showing a rapid increase between the ages of 5 and 20 and a stable rate thereafter

who survive with it and the ratio between numerator and denominator in the living and dead populations will be approximately equal, even though the age structure of the living and dead populations will differ, as we have seen in Chapter 2.

For the purpose of the model, consider an adult population with a prevalence of osteoarthritis of 30%. The model population consists of 500 individuals and osteoarthritis will be allocated amongst 150 of them (30%) by random number generation. We will subject the whole population to death rates of 5–75% and determine which individuals will die by random number generation again. The prevalence of osteoarthritis amongst those who die is determined by counting the number of those amongst the dead population who were allocated the disease in the first stage of the procedure. The estimate of the prevalence of osteoarthritis amongst those who die is determined five times and the results are shown in Table 4.1.

Table 4.1 Modelled prevalence rates for osteoarthritis[a]

Trial	Death rate in population (%)				
	5	10	25	50	75
1	20.0	32.0	29.6	30.4	30.1
2	16.0	46.0	23.2	32.8	31.2
3	20.0	22.0	31.2	26.0	30.9
4	16.0	36.0	36.0	32.4	31.2
5	40.0	32.0	34.4	29.6	30.9
Mean	22.4	33.6	30.9	30.2	30.9
SD	10.0	8.6	5.0	2.7	0.5
SEM	4.9	3.9	2.2	1.2	0.2

[a] $F = 2.15$.

The estimate of the prevalence rate in the live population based on that from the dead population is acceptably reliable for all death rates although it improves at the higher death rates; the standard error of the estimate decreases with increasing death rate, as would be expected. Even with a 5% death rate, however, the estimate, although low, is not significantly different from the expected 30% and there is no significant difference between the mean of the five estimated rates ($F = 2.15$, $p > 0.05$). It is also clear from the table that the best estimate of the living prevalence rate is obtained from the mean of several different studies.

Diseases that Do Contribute towards Death

When we are dealing with diseases that do contribute towards death then prevalence rates in skeletal populations do not approximate to those in the living. I will illustrate this with some modern data for tuberculosis.

From the Registrar General's *Mortality Tables for 1987* we can calculate age-specific prevalence rates which are equivalent to those which would be found in a skeletal population; we can call these the palaeopathological rates[6]. In each ten-year age group the number who die from tuberculosis is divided by the total number of deaths in that age group to give a rate which varies between 0.46 and 0.99 per 10^3. We do not know the prevalence in the living but we can make estimates using some assumptions about the case fatality rate. Let us suppose that it is 10%, that is to say, 10% of those in each age group who contract the disease will die of it. The deaths in each age group thus represent only 10% of the total number with the disease; on this basis, the total number who had the disease can be calculated readily and the prevalence is obtained by dividing this number by the total number alive in the age group. In Figure 4.2 a series of prevalence rates has been calculated with case fatality rates which vary from 1 to 100% and these are compared with the palaeopathological rate. It is evident from this figure that the rates in the living and the dead populations do not agree at all well. With high case fatality rates (which would certainly have applied until recently) the palaeopathological rate seriously overestimates the living rate except in the older age groups, where there is a cross-over when the palaeopathological rate starts to underestimate the living rate. In any past population the death rate from tuberculosis is certain to have been greater than 10% and so the prevalence obtained from skeletal material is likely always to be an underestimate of the living prevalence.

Prevalences in Dead Populations

Having said all this, however, the distinction between diseases which do or do not contribute towards death is important only when projecting prevalences from the dead population to the living, and it is not uncommon for authors to make the assumption that the prevalence of a disease in a group of skeletons directly reflects the experience of the living population of which it was once a part. Age-specific prevalences in skeletal populations can be validly compared so long as we can accept the underlying assumption that the diseases being compared contributed to death in an equal manner in both populations, and this seems reasonable for most eras from which we have skeletons.

As an aside we should note that age-specific prevalences of diseases could *not* legitimately be compared in two populations if there were any reason to suppose that dying from a particular disease affected the site of burial. For example, it might be that at one period of history, individuals with a certain disease were not buried in the usual site, whereas at another period they were. In

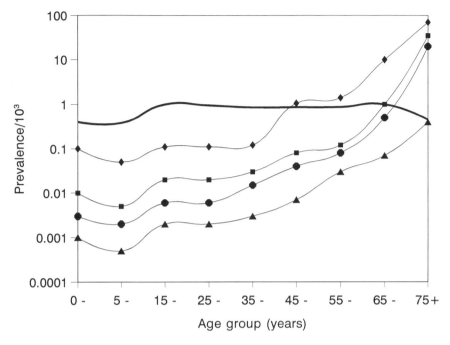

Figure 4.2 Prevalence rates of tuberculosis in living and dead populations based on data from the *Mortality Tables for 1987* of the Registrar General. Note the log scale on the y-axis. Prevalence rates are shown for the dead (palaeopathological) population (thick line) and for living populations with 100% (▲), 20% (●), 10% (■) and 1% (◆) case fatality rates

this case, the age-specific prevalences would vary for reasons which had nothing to do with the frequency of the disease in the living populations.

MISSING DATA

So far the calculation of disease frequency has been discussed as though the skeletons with which we are likely to be dealing are complete, but as everyone who has examined human bones knows, the occasions when this is true are all too few. Small bones, such as those of the hands and feet, are often lost but the disturbance of the grave commonly accounts for damage or loss of the larger elements. This has an important bearing on any sums that are done for calculating prevalence. For example, suppose that we have 120 adult skeletons in 27 of which there is evidence of osteoarthritis of the spine; suppose also that a further 19 have osteoarthritis of the hands and four have osteoarthritis of the hip. The crude prevalence rates would appear to be 225, 158.3 and 33.3 per 10^3 respectively. Suppose, however, that the spines of 17 of the skeletons were too damaged to examine, that 13 lacked hands and that nine had hips missing. How should we represent the prevalence rates knowing this? One way would be to present them as a range of possibilities. If we make the assumption that *none* of the missing joints was affected then we are left with the original rates. On the other hand, if we assume that they were *all* affected then we obtain rates of $(27 + 17)/0.12$, $(19 + 13)/0.12$ and $(4 + 9)/0.12$ per 10^3 for the spine, hands and hip: 366.7, 266.7 and 108.3, respectively. These rates can be thought of as representing the upper limit of the range and the original rates to represent the lower limit. The 'true' rate would thus lie somewhere in-between.

This is a valid if somewhat cumbersome way of going about things and would lead to fearsome problems when trying to attempt any comparative work. An alternative is simply to ignore the missing data, recognising that this would lead to a considerable underestimate of the rate. Or we can make the assumption that the distribution of osteoarthritis amongst the missing joints is similar to that in the joints which *are* present and use the number present minus the number missing as the denominator. Thus the denominators in the example given above now become 103 for the spine, 107 for the hands and 111 for the hips and with these denominators the prevalence rates are now 262.1, 177.6 and 36.0 per 10^3; we might perhaps call these the corrected rates. (All the rates we have discussed so far are shown in Table 4.2 for comparison.)

Of the three methods for dealing with missing data outlined above, the last is to be preferred. There is a final modification which needs to be made, however, when only one of a pair of joints is missing from the assemblage. I can illustrate this with another hypothetical example.

Imagine a population of 115 skeletons, seven of which have osteoarthritis of the hip; the crude (uncorrected) prevalence rate is $7/0.115$, or 60.9 per 10^3. Now suppose that a total of 17 joints is

Table 4.2 Different prevalence rates derived from skeletal populations with missing data[a]

Site	Prevalence rate/10^3		
	Uncorrected crude rate	Uncorrected upper rate	Corrected rate
Spine	225.0	366.7	262.1
Hands	158.3	266.7	177.6
Hip	38.3	108.3	36.0

[a]See text for explanation of rates.

missing; it may be thought that the corrected prevalence rate would be $7/(115 - 7)$, or 71.4 per 10^3, but this is not necessarily so. Let us further suppose that only four skeletons have both hip joints missing and that of the nine lacking only the one, two have osteoarthritis in the joint which *is* present. Thus we have 13 skeletons with one or more hip joints missing, but we know that two of these have osteoarthritis in a least one hip. The total number of skeletons for which we lack any information about the presence of osteoarthritis, therefore, is only 11. The denominator for the prevalence sum is thus 104, and the rate is $7/0.104$, or 67.3 per 10^3. In general terms, then, the denominator for paired joints is the number of skeletons with both joints present, plus the number of single joints (i.e. *one* of the pair) which show evidence of disease.[7]

Disarticulated Material

It is by no means always the case that palaeopathologists have to deal with discrete skeletons, or parts thereof. Investigations are often undertaken on assemblages which consist of a jumbled mass of bones coming from an often completely unknown number of individuals. Faced with such an assemblage, it is custom and practice to calculate a minimum number of individuals (MNI) on the basis of the most frequent anatomical element present, but this figure cannot be used as a denominator for calculating prevalence. It is permissible to use the number of all types of bone, or the number of all one kind of joint as the denominator in the calculation, and the number of affected bones or joints as the numerator.

FURTHER IMPLICATIONS FOR PALAEOPATHOLOGY

What now remains is to discuss the implications of the topics dealt with in this chapter for the interpretation of the results obtained from the examination of skeletons. There are three areas to consider: the nature of the diseases or conditions present in the skeleton; the establishment of *a priori* assumptions against which to test the data; and, lastly, dealing with missing data.

The Nature of Diseases or Conditions

The prevalence of disease in a skeletal population will be a reasonable estimate of the prevalence in the corresponding living population only in those diseases which do not cause death or contribute materially towards it.[8] Thus, when making an inference about the frequency of a disease in a community on the basis of the evidence in their bones it is necessary to know into which category that disease fits. For the disease which occurs most commonly in the skeleton—osteoarthritis—there is not much difficulty although there are some marginal problems. The old lady who is confined to her bed with an arthritic hip or knee and who is immobile is at greater risk of succumbing from hypostatic pneumonia; and in some societies, those who had osteoarthritis to the extent that they could not work, may not have been fed; but there is no point in contemplating these issues too deeply since they have no resolution. As we have seen, there are already too many imperfections inherent in the application of epidemiology to palaeopathology and there is little harm in ignoring some of the more trivial.

We can confidently place the infectious diseases that affect the skeleton into the category of diseases which would have shortened life span directly or indirectly and so their prevalence in the living will be incorrectly estimated, the direction of the error depending upon their case fatality rate. Unfortunately we can have very little idea about what that would have been and can, therefore, only guess at the appropriate correction factor to apply.

In the case of tuberculosis the case fatality rate was likely to have been high until well into the middle of the last century when the number of deaths seems to have decreased well in advance of a knowledge of the true cause of the disease and certainly long before any effective treatments were to hand. Leprosy, by contrast, probably did not have a high mortality rate *per se*, but the associated infections that follow upon anaesthesia of the feet or hands and the social ostracism that was the concomitant of the disease would almost certainly have made the sufferer a poor risk to any primitive insurance society.

Osteomyelitis—the third bone infection which may be seen relatively frequently—stands somewhere between tuberculosis and leprosy, epidemiologically speaking. Long survival times are compatible with the disease but there is a possibility that the infection may spread to other organs or give rise to septicaemia; it may also cause death through renal failure secondary to the production of amyloid.[9]

These few examples show how careful one has to be when projecting skeletal prevalence rates back to the living population and of comparing palaeopathological rates with modern rates; in most cases it is best to consider the two as completely incompatible and reserve any comparisons to other groups of skeletons.

A priori Assumptions

A knowledge of the likely pattern of the prevalence rates of the common diseases which afflict the skeleton will allow the palaeoepidemiologist to generate some *a priori* assumptions with which to test his data. To take a simple case; in any group of adult skeletons, no matter what their provenance, osteoarthritis will be the most common disease. If this is *not* the case, then this suggests that the sample is unusual and that perhaps there is an over-representation of young adults. One constant feature of osteoarthritis is that the prevalence increases considerably with age but that there is not a very great difference in crude prevalence rates between men and women. Consequently if these features are not reflected in the skeletal group under examination, this again suggests that it is unusual in some way. If the expected increase in prevalence with age is not found then this may be the result of errors in the ageing of the skeletons and might indicate that this task should be undertaken by another observer. It goes without saying, of course, that if signs of osteoarthritis are themselves used as ageing criteria age-specific rates are meaningless and, on this account, osteoarthritis should never enter into the reckoning when trying to put an age to a skeleton.

A priori assumptions can be made about other diseases and the genuine palaeoepidemiologist should try to devise as many as possible to apply to his study group. If the number of skeletons is too small to allow valid inferences then it will certainly be too small to allow very much other epidemiological inference no matter how much statistical sleight of hand is indulged in and it would be best to go on to something else, or wait until further data are to hand.

Missing Data

Missing parts bedevil the palaeopathologist's life and it is almost certain that the skeletons which appear to have the most interesting pathology will be missing some key element. To deal with the problem of the incomplete skeleton requires that a tally is kept of the numbers of joints present in an assemblage and not merely the number of individuals since the latter will hardly ever come into use as a denominator. The practical requirement is for some system of record keeping which will quickly and accurately yield both the number of bones present and the number of joints. When presenting prevalence rates to the public it would be nice to think that authors would state how they dealt with missing data and, preferably, what the denominators were in each calculation. If this seems to make the text too tedious, this information could be consigned to an appendix; it would be best to make very strenuous efforts to prevent it from being put on microfiche since this is the most certain way that I know of ensuring that it will never again see the light of day.

NOTES

1. This is a somewhat simplified account. Epidemiologists, however, seem to like nothing more than making simple matters complicated; those who wish for mathematical derivations should consult K.J.

Rothman, *Modern epidemiology*, Boston, Little Brown & Company, 1986, chapter 3.

2. The recommended definitions for the rates which are briefly discussed here are to be found in World Health Organisation, The international classification of diseases and health-related classifications, *World Health Statistics Quarterly*, 1990, 43, 220–23.

3. For further details of fixed and dynamic populations see Rothman, *op cit*, pp 23–9.

4. This is, of course, not true; some cases arise as the result of trauma during adult life and some are secondary to degenerative changes in the spine. These varieties of spondylolysis are by no means as numerous as the childhood cases and we can safely ignore them for the sake of simplicity. Those wishing for further details will find them in G. Amundson, C.C. Edwards and S.R. Garfin, Spondylolisthesis, In: *The spine*, 3rd edition, edited by H.N. Herkowitz, S.R. Garfin, R.A. Balderston, F.J. Eismont, G.R. Bell and S.W. Wiesel, Philadelphia, W.B. Saunders, 1992, pp 913–69.

5. This is also somewhat of a simplification and purists may care to point to the evidence derived from follow-up studies that the lesions do sometimes heal, certainly in unilateral cases. This is gone into more fully elsewhere (T. Waldron, Unilateral spondylolysis, *International Journal of Osteoarchaeology*, 1992, 2, 177–81) but will be resolutely ignored in the present discussion.

6. Registrar General, *Mortality Tables for 1987*, London, HMSO, 1989.

7. To obtain the correct denominators will require the presence or absence of each joint to be recorded; if information is required about the prevalence of disease within the separate compartments of a complex joint—the medial, lateral and patello-femoral compartments of the knee, for example—these will also have to be recorded separately. When reporting the prevalence of disease in complex joints it must be clearly stated whether the data relate to *all* compartments or to its separate components; it is probably best to report a prevalence which relates to all compartments and sub-divide this if necessary. What should *not* be done, since it can be very confusing and defy comparison with other studies, is to devise complicated scoring systems which amalgamate disease if it is present in more than one compartment. Thus if osteoarthritis were found to be present in both the medial and lateral compartments of the same knee, this can *only* be considered as a single case of osteoarthritis—not two—when expressing the prevalence of osteoarthritis of the knee. If authors depart from this practice then the reader may be left wondering just what the rates really mean; see for example P.S. Bridges, Degenerative joint disease in hunter-gatherers and agricul-

turalists from the Southeastern United States, *American Journal of Physical Anthropology*, 1991, 85, 379–91.

8. I am forgetting those other matters which we discussed in Chapter 2 and talking as though we have a representative sample of the whole dead population. Those who wish to complicate things to an overwhelming degree can work out for themselves how they are going to deal with *those*; my guess is that, like good palaeoepidemiologists, they will studiously ignore them.

9. P.A. Revell, *Pathology of bone*, Berlin, Springer, 1986.

5
Comparing Prevalences

One of the more important and interesting problems for the palaeopathologist is to try to make inferences about the changing pattern of disease in the past with a view to suggesting possible causes for any fluctuations which might be observed. This can best be done by comparing disease frequencies between studies but to do this requires a high degree of comparability between different data. The basis of any comparison will be, as we have seen in the previous chapter, prevalence rates, both crude and age-specific.[1] Age-specific rates can be compared between studies but this involves a great many comparisons and there is some advantage in having a single summary rate to describe the experience of an entire population which may then be used for comparative purposes.

The summary prevalence statistic is the crude prevalence rate, but if one tries to use this for comparative purposes a difficulty immediately becomes obvious. For example, Table 5.1 shows age-specific and crude prevalences for a disease in two hypothetical populations, A and B. The crude prevalence rate for A is $390.9/10^3$ and for B, $343.0/10^3$, giving a rate ratio of 1.14 in favour of A. In other words, it would seem that the disease is more common in A than it is in B. Looking at the age-specific rates in columns 3 and 6 of the table, however, this conclusion seems anomalous since, with the exception of the youngest group, they are actually lower in A than in B. Moreover, the population structure in the two populations differs considerably, there being many older individuals in A than in B and many younger individuals in

Table 5.1   Age-specific prevalences of disease in two populations[a]

Age group (years)	A			B		
	N (1)	n (2)	Rate/10^3 (3)	N (4)	n (5)	Rate/10^3 (6)
25–34	32	2	62.5	49	3	61.2
35–44	42	12	266.7	61	20	327.9
45–54	58	27	465.5	30	16	533.3
55+	65	36	553.8	32	20	635.0
Total	197	77	390.9	172	59	343.0

[a] N = Total number in each age group; n = total number affected; crude prevalence for A = $390.0/10^3$ and for B = $343.0/10^3$; rate ratio A:B = 1.14.

B than in A. And herein lies the basis of our problem; the disproportionate number of older individuals in A—in whom the disease is much more common—is artificially elevating the crude prevalence rate. What is needed, then, is some method which will make allowances for the different population structures and produce overall rates which are directly comparable. This is achieved by computing risk or odds ratios or by standardisation; these techniques will be described in what follows.

RISK AND ODDS RATIOS

Suppose that we have two populations with age-specific prevalences $p_1, \ldots p_n$ and $q_1, \ldots q_n$. To compare the prevalences of the two, we could calculate the risk ratios:

$$\frac{p_1}{q_1} \ldots \frac{p_n}{q_n}$$

or the odd ratios:

$$\frac{p_1}{1-p_1} \Bigg/ \frac{q_1}{1-q_1} \ldots \frac{p_n}{1-p_n} \Bigg/ \frac{q_n}{1-q_n}$$

Generally, calculation of the odds ratio (OR) is to be preferred as the age-specific prevalences of many of the common diseases encountered in palaeopathology are likely to vary considerably.[2] The odds ratios of each age stratum can be summed to give a common (or overall) odds ratio ($\hat{OR}$) which relates the age-specific prevalences in two populations in a single figure.[3]

From Table 5.1 the age-specific ORs can be derived as follows. For age 25–34 the ratio is:

$$\frac{62.5}{(1000–62.5)} \Big/ \frac{61.2}{(1000–61.2)} = 1.03$$

For the succeeding age strata, the ORs are: for age 35–44, 0.75; for age 45–54, 0.76; and for age 55+, 0.74.

The common odds ratio is obtained by summing the individual rates thus:

$$\left(\frac{62.5}{937.5}\Big/\frac{61.2}{938.8}\right)+\left(\frac{266.7}{733.3}\Big/\frac{327.9}{672.1}\right)=\left(\frac{465.5}{534.5}\Big/\frac{533.3}{466.7}\right)+\left(\frac{533.8}{466.2}\Big/\frac{625.0}{375.0}\right)$$

which simplifies to:

$$\frac{(62.5 \times 938.8) + (266.7 \times 672.1 + (465.5 \times 466.7) + (533.8 \times 375.0)}{(61.2 \times 937.5) + (327.9 \times 733.3) + (534.5 \times 533.3) + (466.2 \times 625.0)}$$

and becomes:

$$\frac{655\,348}{874\,248} = 0.75$$

From this result it is apparent that the prevalence in population A is actually substantially lower than in B which is just what we would expect from studying the respective age-specific prevalences.[4]

STANDARDISATION

There are two principal methods of standardisation, direct and indirect, and both need to be discussed in some detail.

Direct Standardisation

In this type of standardisation, the age-specific rates of the populations to be compared are applied in turn to a standard population to produce a standardised rate, or comparative mortality figure (CMF). There are several potential choices for the standard population: an entirely artificial population; a real population but entirely unrelated to the populations being compared; or one of the two being compared or a combination of both populations under study. But the choice should not be entirely arbitrary since—as one would expect—consequences follow upon the choice and these may be important.

Let me illustrate the procedure using as the standard the male population of the City of London from the census of 1961[5]. In Table 5.2 the numbers in each of the four age groups corresponding to those in Table 5.1 are shown in column 2 while in columns 3 and 4 the number of cases is derived by multiplying column 2 by the age-specific rates for A and B in columns 3 and 6 of Table 5.1. This yields a total of 1470.9 cases using the rates for A and 1681.2 cases with the rates for B. Thus there are now apparently *more* cases for B than for A and the standardised rate ratio (SRR) is 0.87 in favour of B. Thus, having made allowance for the different population structures we see again that the disease is actually more prevalent in B than in A which is what we expected from an examination of the age-specific rates in Table 5.1. The rate ratio can be analysed statistically as can the difference between two standardised rates.[6]

Table 5.2   Directly standardised prevalences for populations A and B

Age group (years)	N^a	n (rate A)[b]	n (rate B)[c]
25–34	524	32.8	32.1
35–44	599	159.8	196.4
45–54	967	450.1	515.7
55+	1496	828.2	935.0
Total	3586	1470.9	1681.2

N = Total number in each age group in standard population; n = total number affected in each age group calculated from rates for A and B; crude standardised prevalence for A = $410.2/10^3$ and for B = $468.8/10^3$; standardised rate ratio (SRR) A:B = 0.87.
[a] Male population of City of London, 1961.
[b] Obtained from column 3, Table 5.1.
[c] Obtained from column 6, Table 5.1.

It is important to bear in mind that standardised rates are entirely artificial and do not imply anything about the true rates in the original populations except their relationship one to the other. Using a different standard will produce different standardised rates, as can be seen from Table 5.3 where I have substituted for the population of the City of London the male population of the London Borough of Lambeth, again from the 1961 census. Because the population of Lambeth was much larger than that of the City of London, the number of cases is correspondingly greater and the standardised rates are different from those obtained using the City of London standard. In this case they are $375.9/10^3$ for A, and $430.4/10^3$ for B. The SRR, however, is the same as before, 0.87.[7]

Table 5.3 Directly standardised prevalences for populations A and B

Age group (years)	N^a	n (rate A)[b]	n (rate B)[c]
25–34	20 822	1301.4	1274.3
35–44	25 134	6703.2	8241.4
45–54	25 870	12 042.5	13 796.5
55+	39 088	21 646.9	24 430.0
Total	110 914	41 694.0	47 742.2

N = Total number in each age group in standard population; n = total number affected in each age group calculated from rates for A and B; crude standardised prevalence for A = $375.9/10^3$ and for B = $430.4/10^3$; standardised rate ratio (SRR) A:B = 0.87.
[a]Male population of London Borough of Lambeth, 1961.
[b]Obtained from column 3, Table 5.1.
[c]Obtained from column 6, Table 5.1.

As I have said earlier, it is permissible to use one of the original populations or a combination of both as the standard and this might be the most convenient thing to do on occasion. Using the combined populations of A and B as the standard produces the results shown in Table 5.4; again the standardised rates are different but the SRR once more comes out to 0.87 showing that the arithmetic is right. (For comparison, the crude prevalence rate and the various standardised rates are shown in Table 5.5.)

Table 5.4   Directly standardised prevalences for populations A and B

Age group (years)	N^a	n (rate A)[b]	n (rate B)[c]
25–34	81	5.1	5.0
35–44	103	27.5	33.8
45–54	88	41.0	46.9
55+	97	53.7	60.6
Total	369	127.3	146.3

N = Total number in each age group in standard population derived from A + B; n = total number affected in each age group calculated from rates for A and B; crude standardised prevalence for A = $345.0/10^3$ and for B = $396.5/10^3$.
[a] Combined populations of A + B.
[b] Obtained from column 3, Table 5.1.
[c] Obtained from column 6, Table 5.1.

Table 5.5   Summary of prevalences obtained for populations A and B with different standards

Prevalence	A	B	Standardised rate ratio A:B
Crude	390.0	343.0	1.14
City of London	410.2	468.8	0.87
A + B	343.0	396.5	0.87
London Borough of Lambeth	375.9	430.4	0.87

Standardisation then gives a means of comparing two populations directly and the choice of standard seems largely irrelevant. And that *is* the case until one comes to make inter-study comparisons. For example, suppose that population A had been studied by one investigator who published standardised rates based on the City of London and that population B had been studied by another investigator using Lambeth. We now have the situation where the standardised rate for A is given as $410.2/10^3$ while for B it is given as $430.4/10^3$. If we were now to compare these rates, the SRR would be 410.2/430.4 or 0.95. No combination of rates other than those in which both A and B are standardised to the same standard will give us the correct answer. This brings out the important point that standardised rates cannot be compared unless the same standard has been used; this may seem an obvious point to labour but it is one which may be forgotten.

For other than inter-study comparisons in palaeoepidemiology, then, a common standard should be used and it seems highly doubtful that one could be agreed on without the deliberations of an expert committee or two but I would suggest that agreement should come sooner rather than later.[8]

Indirect Standardisation

Indirect standardisation in a sense reverses the procedure followed in the direct method. In this case the age-specific rates from a standard population are applied to the population under study to produce what are called expected numbers of cases. The number of expected cases in each age group is summed and compared with the number observed to produce a standardised mortality (or morbidity) ratio, or SMR. The SMR is thus derived as:[9]

$$SMR = \frac{Observed}{Expected} \times 100$$

The procedure is illustrated in Table 5.6 with our old friends A and B. On this occasion the age-specific rates from a standard population, shown in column 1 of the table, are applied to each of the age groups in turn to obtain the expected numbers shown in columns 4 and 7; the observed numbers are shown in the preceding columns. For A the total number expected is 80.7 and the total observed is 77; for B the figures are 57.0 and 59, respectively. The SMR for A is thus 95.8 and for B it is 103.5; the ratio between these two standard rates is 0.93. For each SMR a 95% confidence interval (CI) can be determined and an estimate made as to whether the difference between the two SMRs is statistically significant.[10]

Notice that although this method of standardisation has a similar effect to the direct method in producing a standardised rate which is lower for A than for B, the ratio between the two standardised rates is different because neither the rates nor the populations to which they are applied are the same as in the direct method.

In modern epidemiology the indirect method is used much more frequently than the direct, particularly in occupational epidemiology where the effects of exposure to harmful materials are being assessed.[11] Since the aim in these studies is most frequently to see

Table 5.6   Indirect standardisation of populations A and B[a]

Age group (years)	Prevalence/10^3 (1)	A N (2)	A O (3)	A E (4)	B N (5)	B O (6)	B E (7)
25–34	50.1	32	2	1.6	49	3	2.5
35–44	375.6	42	12	15.8	61	20	22.9
45–54	424.8	58	27	24.6	30	16	12.7
55+	591.4	65	36	38.4	32	20	18.9
Total			77	80.7		59	57.0

N = Total number in each age group (from Table 5.1); O = number of cases observed (from Table 5.1); E = number of cases expected; standardised mortality ratio for A (SMR_A) = 77/80.4 = 95.8; SMR_B = 59/57 = 103.5; standardised rate ratio (SRR) = 0.93.

how much an exposed population varies from normal, great care is taken in deciding which standard rates to use. Often it is the sex- and age-specific rates which applied in the general population at the time the study was undertaken. Where local rates are available these may be used in preference. What is important is that unless the same rates are used in different studies, then inter-study comparisons will be invalid and even when the same rates *are* used, it may still not be valid to compare SMRs directly, although one will frequently see this done in the literature where league tables of SMRs are often compiled to show the supposed relative effects of an exposure on different populations.[12]

What is frequently overlooked by those who use the indirect method is that the age structure of the populations being compared affects the calculation of the expected numbers and if it is markedly different in the two then an erroneous impression will be gained. I can illustrate this with a simple example shown in Table 5.7. Here we have two populations, C and D, with identical age-specific prevalence rates in two sub-groups, young and old, but with greatly different numbers in each of the two groups. The rates in the standard population (S), shown in column 3 of the table, are applied to each of the sub-groups in turn to obtain the expected numbers, which are 7.5 and 90 for C and 45 and 15 for D. The SMRs are obtained as follows:

Table 5.7 Indirect standardisation of two populations[a]

	Standard (S)			C			D		
	N	n	P	N	n	P	N	n	P
Young	2000	30	15	500	9	18	3000	54	18
Old	6000	180	30	3000	150	50	500	25	50
Total	9000	210	23.3	3500	159	45.4	3500	79	22.6

[a]N = Total number in age group; n = total number of cases; P = prevalence/10^3; standardised mortality ratio for C (SMR_C) = 159/97.5 = 163.1; SMR_D = 79/60 = 131.7; By direct standardisation on population S, standardised rate for C = D = 37.3; standardised rate ratio (SRR) = 1.

$$SMR_C = \frac{(9 + 150)}{(7.5 + 90)} = \frac{159}{97.5} \times 100 = 163.1$$

and

$$SMR_D = \frac{(54 + 25)}{(45 + 15)} = \frac{79}{60} \times 100 = 131.7.$$

These results suggest that the disease is more common in C than in D, which is obviously incorrect as the age-standardised rates are the same in the two populations; the anomaly results from the difference in the age distributions. If the rates are standardised directly to population S, then the standardised rate for both C and D is 37.3 and the SRR is unity, which is what the age-specific rates would have led us to believe in the first instance.

The lesson is that SMRs cannot be directly compared unless the age structure of the populations being compared is very similar or unless age-specific SMRs are compared;[13] this is rather a cumbersome procedure, however, and most investigators prefer to work with a summary measure.

A problem that will be of particular relevance to palaeoepidemiology is which rates to use for indirect standardisation? In any kind of morbidity study this is a source of difficulty but there is a simple solution, and this is to use the combined age-specific prevalence rates of the two populations combined. This has been done for populations A and B in Table 5.8 which shows the combined rates and the observed and expected numbers. The

Table 5.8   Indirect standardisation using combined prevalences[a]

Age group (years)	Prevalence/10^3 for A + B	A		B	
		O	E	O	E
25–34	61.7	2	2.0	3	3.0
35–44	213.6	12	9.0	20	13.0
45–54	488.6	27	28.3	16	14.7
55+	577.3	36	37.5	20	18.5
Total		77	76.8	59	49.2

[a] O = Number of cases observed; E = number of cases expected; standardised mortality ratio for A (SMR_A) = 77/76.8 = 100.3; SMR_B = 59/49.2 = 119.9; standardised rate ratio SRR = 0.84.

SMR for A now becomes 100.3 and for B, 119.9. These are different from those computed earlier and the rate ratio is 0.84.[14]

WHICH METHOD OF COMPARISON TO USE?

The odds ratio method is probably the best to use to compare prevalences between populations. The common odds ratio provides a simple summary statistic which expresses the differences between two populations in a manner which is readily understood. Where three (or more) populations are to be compared, a common odds ratio can be compared between the first and the second, the first and the third, and so on; in effect, this is using the first population as a kind of standard population.

The indirect method of standardisation is overwhelmingly the most popular amongst modern epidemiologists but it has come in for a lot of criticism over the years. As long ago as 1923 Wolfenden declared that 'it should be substituted for the direct method ... only after due examination' and Yule noted in 1934 that it was safe 'only for the comparison of single pairs of populations'.[15] Nothing daunted by these early caveats, epidemiologists continue to use SMRs inappropriately despite warnings by more recent critics such as Rothman who declares that 'a common standard should be employed, and comparison of SMRs should be avoided.'[16]

To some extent the problem of which rate to use is solved in palaeoepidemiology; there are to my knowledge no published rates for the prevalence of disease in skeletal populations which could be used to standardise study populations and there are precious few easily available for modern populations.[17] As we have seen, however, SMRs can be computed from the combined rates of the two populations under study but they cannot be directly compared with those given by other workers.

The direct method, on the other hand, has two advantages. Any population, real or imaginary, can be taken for the standard and, so long as the same standard is used, comparisons can be made directly between studies. There is one drawback with the direct method which has not so far been mentioned, however, and this deserves a quick note. Where the number of individuals in a sub-group is small, the prevalence rate can appear to be very high if one or two cases are present. Where it seems likely that a high prevalence rate is the result of small numbers in the base population, then it would be prudent either to wait until the number can be enhanced through the examination of more skeletons or combine age classes. With this proviso, I recommend the direct method as that of choice in palaeoepidemiology if the odds ratio method is not to be used.

A Cautionary Note

Summing odds ratios or calculating standardised prevalences has one disadvantage which should be mentioned and this relates to a potential *loss* of information. For example, it may be the case that a disease is equally prevalent in the younger age groups, of two populations but substantially different in the older groups, and although this will be reflected in the common odds ratio or in the SRR, there will be no information as to where the difference arises. In another case, a disease may be substantially higher in the younger age group of one population but substantially lower in the older group compared with that against which it is being compared. The common odds ratio or the SRR may thus be close to unity, totally obscuring some extremely interesting differences. On this account it may be best always to compare age-specific ORs as well as the common odds ratio, providing that the sample sizes in the different age groups are sufficient to provide a reliable estimate.

NOTES

1. It has already been said that prevalence is not strictly a rate but this usage is so common that it seems perverse not to follow it here.
2. For further discussion of risk and odds ratios see H.A. Kahn and C.T. Sempos, *Statistical methods in epidemiology*, New York, Oxford University Press, 1989.
3. The calculation of the common odds ratio is derived from N. Mantel and W. Haenszel, Statistical aspects of the analysis of data from retrospective studies of disease, *Journal of the National Cancer Institute*, 1959, 22, 719–48. Further details about this method of comparing prevalences can be found in D. Clayton and M. Hills, *Statistical methods in epidemiology*, Oxford, Oxford University Press, 1993, Chapters 14 and 15.
4. The 95% confidence intervals can be calculated to give a measure of the significance of the common odds ratio; in this case they are 0.68–0.83.
5. This was chosen because I had been using it for some other purpose and it was sufficiently small not to give ridiculously large numbers of 'cases'. The data were originally published in *Census 1961, England and Wales*, London, HMSO, 1966.
6. For the calculation of 95% confidence intervals see M.J. Gardner and D.G. Altman, *Statistics with confidence*, London, BMJ, 1989, pp 59–61. The significance of the difference between rates can be measured using Cochran's test; see P. Armitage and G. Berry, *Statistical methods in medical research*, 2nd edition, Oxford, Blackwell, 1987, pp 399–405. A more mathematical treatment of standardisation is given by K.J. Rothman, *Modern epidemiology*, Boston, Little Brown & Co, 1986, chapter 5.
7. Although it seems intuitive that the SRR will remain constant since the number of cases is determined by the age-specific rates of the populations being compared, this is actually *not* so and the present example may appear to be somewhat misleading in this respect.
8. In fact the City of London population shown here could be used. That it is a population of males and that standardisation procedures might be carried out on a population of female skeletons matters not a whit.
9. Although it is usual for the result of the divison sum to be multiplied by 100, readers may note instances in the literature where this convention is not followed.

10. Gardner and Altman, *op cit*, pp 59–62. To test if an individual SMR differs significantly from 100 a chi-squared test with 1 degree of freedom can be used where $\chi^2 = (\text{Observed} - \text{Expected})^2/(\text{Expected})$. (For further details see H. Checkoway, N.E. Pearce and D.J. Crawford-Brown, *Research methods in occupational epidemiology*, New York, Oxford University Press, 1989, p 127, or Armitage and Berry, *op cit*, pp 400–1.)

11. For occupational examples see Checkoway et al, *op cit*, and R.R. Monson, *Occupational epidemiology*, Boca Raton, CRC Press, 1990.

12. Rothman, *op cit*, has some pungent words to say about this habit; see especially p 48.

13. See Checkoway et al, *op cit*, p 126.

14. Note that the indirect SRRs are not the same, whereas the direct SRRs are. This is because the application of different standard rates to the same population will produce different expected numbers and hence different SMRs.

15. H.H. Wolfenden, On the methods of comparing the mortalities of two or more communities, and the standardization of death rates, *Journal of the Royal Statistical Society*, 1923, 86, 399–411; G. Yule, On some points relating to vital statistics, more especially statistics of occupational mortality, *ibid*, 97, 1–84.

16. Rothman, *op cit*, p 49.

17. I have calculated some prevalence rates for osteoarthritis for skeletal populations from a number of different sites in England. They range in time from Anglo-Saxon to the middle of the 18th century and are shown in the table below:

Age-specific prevalence rates ($/10^3$) for osteoarthritis in a palaeopathological population

	Males	Females
25–34	44.9	41.7
35–44	333.3	246.4
45+	455.3	373.9
Total	300.9	210.0

6
Analytical Epidemiology

A distinction is sometimes made between descriptive methods in epidemiology, such as the determination of incidence and prevalence, and analytical methods in which hypotheses are said to be tested. There is very little to justify this separation of methods and Rothman in particular has some rather harsh words to say on the matter.[1] Irrespective of one's personal feelings, however, this distinction is probably here to stay and I have bowed to convention by discussing some methods under this heading.

There is a somewhat limited opportunity to use analytical methods in palaeoepidemiology but this is probably all the more reason for using those which we do have and I will try to illustrate some in what follows. I shall discuss principally the case-control study and some methods of measuring differences between frequencies of disease using odds and risk ratios.

THE CASE-CONTROL STUDY

The case-control study has a number of attractions to the epidemiologist. It is relatively cheap, it can be completed much more quickly than a longitudinal study, and it is particularly useful for studying rare diseases. In modern epidemiology it is most often used to ascertain the part which various exposures and activities play in the aetiology of disease.[2] The way in which a case-control study is undertaken is rather the reverse of the cohort study. In the latter, one begins with an exposure or some other event and

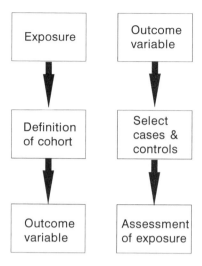

Figure 6.1 Outline of different strategies adopted in prospective or cross-sectional studies (left) and case-control studies (right)

then goes on to measure an outcome variable. In a case-control study, the starting point is the outcome and then one seeks retrospectively to determine the event or exposures which produced this outcome (Figure 6.1). The study group in the case-control study are the cases which have been selected as fulfilling certain entry criteria, perhaps all adult males who developed acute myeloid leukaemia in a five-year period. The entry criteria must be elaborated before there is any selection of cases and these should be strictly adhered to; it is surprising how often entry criteria are relaxed when it is seen how difficult it is to recruit a sufficient number of cases into the study! A criterion might be, for example, that the diagnosis has been agreed by a panel of three (or whatever number) pathologists; another might be that the patients should all be living, all male, and so on.

Having drawn the cases, the controls are selected so that they are as like the cases as possible, except that, by definition, they do not have the disease under study. In fact, this may lead to a degree of 'over-matching' with loss of useful information, and the selection of controls is nowadays rather less constrained than was formerly the case.[3]

Once both cases and controls have been selected, then one moves into the next stage of the procedure which is to determine what events or exposures they might all have experienced. This is usually done by means of a questionnaire or interview. The nature of the questionnaire will depend upon the investigator's preconceived notions of the causation of the disease in question and this obviously *has* to be so, since the likelihood of an individual completing a questionnaire is inversely related to its length; a questionnaire which tries to be all-inclusive and which runs to several pages is very much less likely to be taken seriously than one which asks a few simple, direct questions. In the example of myeloid leukaemia, the investigator might be interested to know how many of the individuals in the study had exposure to radiation or to organic solvents or to pesticides. He will do this most often by asking for a detailed occupational history using the various job titles as surrogates of exposure. In some studies it may be possible to supplement this information by actual measures of exposure from which a dose–response effect might be obtained but this happens much less frequently than one would like.

At some point, the investigator will have information on how many cases and how many controls fall into each exposure group; so many may have been working in jobs which involved exposure to radiation, to solvents, to pesticides and so on. The trick now is to see whether there is any difference in the numbers exposed amongst the cases than amongst the controls and, if so, whether this difference is statistically significant; this is all achieved using the chi-squared (χ^2) test. Suppose that in the leukaemia study there were 200 cases and 200 controls and that 27 of the cases had exposure to organic solvents whereas only 11 of the controls did. The results are presented in a simple tabular form as shown in Table 6.1 from which it can be shown that $\chi^2 = 7.43$ with 1 degree of freedom and that $p < 0.01$. This is a highly significant result (statistically) and would certainly be leapt upon by the investigator to show that exposure to solvents was highly likely to lead to the development of leukaemia or at least form the basis of his next grant application.

Table 6.1 Number of cases and controls with exposure to solvents[a]

	Exposure	No exposure	Total
Cases	27	173	200
Controls	11	189	200
Total	38	362	400

[a] $\chi^2 = 7.43, p < 0.01$.

Confounding

One of the issues which must be considered in a case-control study is that of confounding. A confounding factor is one which may produce the same outcome variable as the exposure being studied[4] and unless account is taken of it in the analysis of the results, false conclusions may be drawn. In any study of lung cancer, for example, smoking would be a potential confounding factor and cases and controls would either have to be matched for smoking habit or smoking would have to be allowed for in the statistical analysis. There are a number of ways in which confounding can be allowed for but one which is commonly used and which would suit almost all palaeoepidemiological applications is the Mantel-Haenszel chi-squared procedure.[5]

Let us suppose that in our solvents and leukaemia study we had found from our questionnaire data that a substantial number of individuals had been X-rayed and we felt that the radiation they had received might also be a possible cause of their leukaemia. We could stratify the data to take account of this, and this has been done in Table 6.2. Of the cases, 29 have had doses of X-rays whereas this is true for only five of the controls. Using the Mantel-Haenszel procedure, $\chi^2 = 3.47$, which is a non-significant result and we can see that, having allowed for the radiation exposure, there is no significant difference between the cases and controls with respect to their solvent status.

The Odds Ratio

In addition to analysing the results of a case-control study by the use of χ^2, the odds ratio can also be calculated. This is an estimate

Table 6.2 Number of cases and controls with exposure to solvents and X-rays[a]

	Exposure	No exposure	Total
Cases			
X-rays	11	18	29
No X-rays	16	155	171
Controls			
X-rays	0	5	5
No X-rays	11	184	195
	200	200	400

[a] $\chi^2 = 3.47$ (not significant).

of the risk associated with a particular exposure and in some texts it may still be referred to as the relative risk.[6] The basis of the calculation is shown in Table 6.3 where the cells bear the same relationship to each other as in the two earlier tables. The odds ratio is calculated simply as:

$$\text{Odds ratio} = \frac{ad}{be}$$

The odds ratio can be calculated separately from the Mantel-Haenszel χ^2 or there are a number of computer programs which will calculate χ^2 , the odds ratio and its 95% confidence intervals (CI) in one go. In Table 6.1 the odds ratio is 2.68 and CI = 1.29–5.57; in Table 6.2 the odds ratio is 2.07 and CI = 0.96–4.48. In the first example the CI does not include unity whereas in the second it does so; the first would be considered statistically significant but not the second.

Table 6.3 Odds ratio in a case-control study[a]

	Exposed		Total
	Yes	No	
Cases	a	b	a + b
Controls	c	d	c + d
Total	a + c	b + d	a + b + c + d

[a] The odds ratio is given as ad/bc.

THE CASE CONTROL STUDY IN PALAEOEPIDEMIOLOGY

As I mentioned at the start of this chapter, the use of the case-control study in palaeopathology is somewhat restricted by the nature of the material with which we have to deal but that should only encourage its use where it can be helpful. In palaeoepidemiology the case-control approach could be used to test associations between conditions, or to test the proposition that a disease may be more common in one group than another.

There have been rather few examples of case-control studies applied to palaeoepidemiology but I can illustrate the first example mentioned above with a study of my own and supply some hypothetical data to an observed association for the second.

In the clinical literature there are several instances in which spondylolysis of spondylolisthesis has been found in association with spina bifida occulta; the proportion of those with spondylolysis in whom spina bifida also occurs has been quoted to be in the range of 13–70%.[7] There is also some evidence that the prevalence of transitional vertebrae is lower in patients with spondylolysis than in controls. These lesions are all readily identified in the skeleton, and as none is all that common, a case-control approach is well suited to study the reported associations.

To be included in the study we are examining here, skeletons with spondylolysis were required to have an intact sacrum so that the presence or absence of spina bifida and transitional vertebrae could be established. Sixty-four cases were found from different archaeological sites. All were adults and for each case two controls were chosen at random from amongst the remaining adult skeletons at the appropriate site which did *not* have spondylolysis. No matching was made but allowance was made for sex in the analysis.

The results of the study are shown in Tables 6.4 and 6.5. Amongst the cases, 43 were male and 21 female; the corresponding numbers amongst the controls were 79 and 49, respectively. Five of the cases had spina bifida, as did nine of the controls; the odds ratio was 1.10 and CI = 0.30–3.90.

Table 6.4 Number of cases and controls with spina bifida[a]

		Spina bifida	
		+	−
Cases	Male	4	39
	Female	1	20
Controls	Male	6	73
	Female	3	46

[a]Odds ratio 1.10, 95% CI = 0.35–3.44.

Table 6.5 Number of cases and controls with transitional vertebrae[a]

		Transitional vertebrae	
		+	−
Cases	Male	2	41
	Female	0	21
Controls	Male	9	70
	Female	2	47

[a]Odds ratio 0.32, 95% CI = 0.07–1.50.

Only two of the cases had transitional vertebrae, compared with eleven of the referents. In this case the odds ratio was 0.35 and CI = 0.07–1.50; another non-significant result.

This study therefore failed to show the expected increase in the prevalence of spina bifida in the cases with spondylolysis or to demonstrate that they had a lower prevalence of transitional vertebrae for reasons which do not need to be considered further. It does show the case-control study in action, however, and demonstrates its economy.[8]

For the second example, let us suppose that we wish to examine the suggestion that diffuse idiopathic skeletal hyperostosis (DISH) is particularly common in those following the religious way of life or otherwise of 'high status'. A good deal of evidence is accumulating that this is actually the case and some reasons have been suggested. On a number of monastic sites it has been found that the prevalence of DISH is higher than expected amongst the monks; it is also a common observation that burials within a church—an indication of 'high status'—have a higher prevalence of DISH than those buried in the cemetery outside.[9] Let us say that we have 43 cases of DISH, all males, and that we choose two controls at random from the remaining adult males and then see how many might reasonably be said to be monks or clerics or of 'high status' using criteria decided upon at the start of the study. The findings are set out in Table 6.6. Here we can see that 18 of the cases were high status compared with only seven of the controls, giving a χ^2 of 20.70 an odds ratio of 8.13 and a CI = 3.04–21.70, which is all highly significant and confirms our view that the association is not likely to have arisen by chance.

Table 6.6 Results of a case-control study of diffuse idiopathic skeletal hyperostosis (DISH) and social status[a]

	Religious/ high status	Low status	Total
Case	18	25	43
Control	7	79	86
Total	25	104	129

[a] χ^2 = 20.70, p <0.001. Odds ratio = 8.13, CI = 3.04–21.70.

SAMPLE SIZES AND POWER OF A STUDY

The object of analytical methods in epidemiology is to test a hypothesis; formally this is the null hypothesis which states that there is *no* difference between cases and controls, for example. Statistical methods are used to test the null hypothesis; if it is rejected then one is entitled to suggest some other hypothesis which is considered plausible (at least by the investigator) to explain the facts.[10] There are two errors which the unwary may commit, however; a true null hypothesis may not be rejected, giving a false positive result; alternatively, the null hypothesis may fail to be rejected when it is not actually true, giving a false negative result. These errors are referred to as Type I and Type II, respectively. The degree of confidence with which the null hypothesis can be rejected is expressed through a test of significance from which a p value is obtained; the lower the value of p, the more confident we can be that a Type I error is not being committed. The confidence with which one can be certain that one is not accepting a false null hypothesis is expressed through the power of the study. It is possible to specify the desired power of a study and use this to calculate sample sizes.

The calculation of the numbers required in a case-control study depends: upon the magnitude of the difference which one wishes to detect between cases and controls (5%, 10% and so on); the significance level (referred to in this calculation as α), which is generally set at 5%; and the required power of the study (ß), which may typically be 80%. The calculations are somewhat tedious and the equations and tables required are to be found explained in detail elsewhere;[11] there is no simple method.

Having carried out a study which has a negative outcome it may be helpful to determine whether it was actually powerful enough to reject a false null hypothesis. Increasing the number of controls increases the power of a study and this is a useful device in any study if it is feasible. The procedure for calculating the power of a study is similar to that for estimating required numbers: the equations are the same but different terms are unknown. Those wishing to carry out the calculations are again referred to the book by Kelsey and her colleagues.[11]

RELATIVE RISK

Relative risk—as intimated above—is closely related to the odds ratio and is the comparison of the incidence or prevalence of a disease in two groups of individuals who are similar except for the presence or absence of some factor under investigation. For example, if the prevalence rate in a group possessing or exposed to the factor is p_1 and the prevalence amongst the unexposed is p_2, then the relative risk (RR) is given as:

$$RR = \frac{p_1}{p_2}$$

In many cases the relative risk closely approximates the odds ratio. For example, consider a control group which has a prevalence for some condition of $12/10^5$ and a study group in which the prevalence is $70/10^5$. The relative risk is $70/12 = 5.83$ and the odds ratio is $(70 \times 99\ 988)/(12 \times 99\ 930) = 5.84$. The difference between the relative risk and the odds ratio increases as the incidence or prevalence of the condition under consideration increases; for rare conditions they will very often show no sensible difference.

The relative risk can be calculated in palaeoepidemiology using prevalence data instead of the odds ratio. For instance, in the study of DISH we discussed earlier, suppose the prevalence in the high status population was 8.4% and in the control group it was 3.6%, then the relative risk is 2.33 with a 95% CI of 1.59–3.41.

When dealing with the common diseases, calculating the relative risk is a perfectly reasonable approach, but with more rare disorders, calculating the odds ratio through a case-control study is to be preferred.

THE MORBIDITY ODDS RATIO

In 1981, Miettinen and Wang[12] introduced the mortality odds ratio (MOR) as an alternative to the proportional mortality ratio (PMR) about which they had some reservations: firstly that it was not, they argued, a quantity of intrinsic interest, being used only as a surrogate for the desired number of cases observed/number of cases expected (O/E ratio) from which a standardised mortality ratio (SMR) could be computed; and secondly, because the PMR is dependent upon how common other causes of death are relative to the disease of interest. To supplant the PMR they proposed the mortality odds ratio, which they considered was more useful, being analogous to the odds ratio in a case-control study.

The calculation is the same as for the odds ratio in a case-control study. The number of cases whose cause of death is the object of the study is determined in each of two groups (exposed and non-exposed, for example) and the number of all other causes of death is also established. In a hypothetical case we might obtain the results as set out in Table 6.7. The proportional mortality in the exposed group is $(18/94) = 0.19$, while in the non-exposed group it is $(6/149) = 0.04$. The PMR $= (0.19/0.04) = 4.75$. The MOR (ad/bc) $= (18 \times 143)/(6 \times 76) = 5.64$.

Table 6.7   Results of a hypothetical proportional mortality study[a]

Cause of death	Exposed	Non-exposed
Disease of interest	18 (*a*)	6 (*b*)
All other diseases	76 (*c*)	143 (*d*)
Proportional mortality	0.19	0.04

[a]Proportional mortality ratio (PMR) = 0.19/0.04 = 4.75; mortality odds ratio (MOR) = $ad/bc = 2574/456 = 5.64$.

We cannot calculate the *mortality* odds ratio in palaeoepidemiology but it is feasible to adapt it to calculate a *morbidity* odds ratio with which the frequency of a disease could be compared in two groups. I published an illustrative example looking at the frequency of spondylolysis in two groups.[13] In the first there were 10 cases of spondylolysis and 466 other conditions; in the second the corresponding figures were 13 and 231 (see Table 6.8). The MOR was 0.38 with a 95% CI = 0.17–0.88, suggesting that spondylolysis was significantly less common in the first group than the second.

Table 6.8   Spondylolysis in different skeletal groups[a]

	Group 1	Group 2
Spondylolysis	10	13
All other conditions	466	231

[a]Mortality odds ratio (MOR) = 0.38, 95% CI = 0.17–0.88.

Calculating the MOR seems about as simple and straightforward a procedure as can be imagined but some thought has to be given to deciding exactly what constitutes a 'disease' or 'condition' for entry into the equation as '*c*' and '*d*'. There is no difficulty in including examples of gross pathology but with many conditions there is no dichotomous state of 'present' or 'absent'; do minute osteophytes or a tiny trace of periosteal new bone count as disease? And is one counting all different conditions, in which case the number could conceivably be greater than the number of skeletons present, or simply the number of diseased skeletons?

In practice the differentiation between normal and abnormal tends to be somewhat arbitrary and will differ from one observer to another. So long as the strategy adopted for distinguishing abnormal from normal is codified before starting the study, a disease will be as defined by the rule laid down and the analysis should be valid. And it is the number of conditions and not diseased skeletons which should be counted.

Missing data may cause problems but only if the preservation of the two groups differs substantially. If it does not, then it is probably permissible to make the assumption that any loss of information will tend to balance out and that there is no bias in the study. This will require some preliminary assessment of the state of preservation and if there are good reasons to suppose that it is markedly disparate between the groups, this would suggest that one would be more fruitfully employed doing something else.

NOTES

1. K.J. Rothman, *Modern epidemiology*, Boston, Little Brown & Co, 1986, pp xii–xiii.
2. See J.J. Schlesselman, *Case control studies. Design, conduct, analysis.* New York, Oxford University Press, 1982 for the most thorough account of this kind of study. Incidentally, it is now fashionable to refer to these studies as case-referent, rather than case-control studies to reflect the rather less emphasis on very tight matching nowadays. There is little harm in adhering to the older, more familiar nomenclature, however.
3. For overmatching, see Schlesselman, *op cit*, pp 109–11; Rothman, *op cit*, pp 247–9.
4. Strictly speaking a confounder should satisfy two conditions: (i) it is a risk factor for the disease under study and (ii) it is associated with the study exposure but is not a consequence of it. In practice, any other risk factor which is not itself a consequence of exposure may be regarded as a confounder and it is in the restricted sense that the term is used here. For further details see Schlesselman, *op cit*, pp 58–63.
5. I do not propose to go into the technicalities of this or of other procedures to deal with confounding. Those who wish to find out more should consult the original paper of N. Mantel and W. Haenszel,

Statistical aspects of the analysis of data from retrospective studies of disease, *Journal of the National Cancer Institute*, 1959, 22, 719–748, or Schlesselman, *op cit*, pp 183–90; 254–63; 275–80.

6. The relative risk is estimated from a prevalence or incidence study and strictly speaking should not be used when referring to the results of a case-control study; in the latter the odds ratio is the preferred statistic.

7. The references to the papers containing these observations and others mentioned in this section can be found in my paper, A case-referent study of spondylolysis and spina bifida and transitional vertebrae in human skeletal remains, *International Journal of Osteoarchaeology*, 1993, 3, 55–7.

8. The economy of effort can be appreciated by comparing the amount of work needed to examine the association between spondylolysis and spina bifida using the cross-sectional method. In this case, all the individual skeletons have to be examined to determine which have the conditions. In the case-control study we need only know the cases with spondylolysis (or a random sub-sample of them if the numbers are sufficiently great) and examine them and the relatively small number of controls.

9. To date little of this evidence has been formally published, but see T. Waldron, DISH at Merton Priory: evidence for a "new" occupational disease? *British Medical Journal*, 1985, 291, 1762–3.

10. Authors are particularly adept at devising biologically plausible explanations for associations which they find in epidemiological studies, many of which may actually be due to the operation of confounders. This has been discussed in two interesting papers: G.D. Smith and A.N. Phillips, Confounding in epidemiological studies: why "independent" effects may not be all that they seem, *British Medical Journal*, 1992, 305, 757–9 and G.D. Smith, A.N. Phillips and J.D. Neaton, Smoking as an "independent" risk factor for suicide: illustration of an artifact from observational epidemiology? *Lancet*, 1992, 340, 709–12.

11. J.L. Kelsey, W.D. Thompson and A.S. Evans, *Methods in observational epidemiology*, New York, Oxford University Press, 1986, pp 271–8. There are plenty of other references to the calculation of power and sample sizes but this is the one which I have found most straightforward and the easiest to follow.

12. O.S. Miettinen and J.-D. Wang, An alternative to the proportionate mortality ratio, *American Journal of Epidemiology*, 1981, 114, 144–8.

13. T. Waldron, Variations in the rates of spondylolysis in early populations, *International Journal of Osteoarchaeology*, 1991, 1, 63–5.

7
A Guide to Best Practice

Throughout the book I have issued several warnings and made some recommendations as to what I consider to be 'best practice'. This chapter will try to synthesise all these into a cohesive whole. At the outset there is a distinction to be made between studies which report new data and those in which comparisons are to be made using data already published.

For the first kind of study, reporting new data, it is preferable (if not absolutely obligatory) that the author undertakes all the preliminary work himself, or if this cannot be done, for reasons of time or scale, for example, then he should ensure that all those working on the project are reporting consistently. The best way to make sure that this is indeed the case is for all those involved to make some independent determinations—of age, sex and pathology, for example—on a sub-sample of the population and compare results. Any marked differences must be reconciled and the exercise continued until a satisfactory level of agreement is reached.[1] It is often a salutary lesson for a single observer to re-examine the same skeletons again after an interval of a few days or weeks and compare the notes made on the two occasions; but let us not be too gloomy.

The absolute numbers of each age and sex group should be given in the account of the findings, as should the numbers in which disease is certainly present, certainly absent and unknown. For comparative purposes it is essential that the same age classes are used; one simply cannot compare two populations if one is stratified in ten-year age groups and the other is classified as 'young', 'middle-aged' and 'old'. It seems entirely reasonable to attempt some broad age classification and it is interesting to hear from forensic anthropologists that they are confident in their ability to do so; palaeopathologists also should be. What is essential, however, is that the criteria used for the attribution of age and sex should be stated; given the constraints on space imposed on authors by most editors, all that may be allowed is reference to the methods, but this should always be the minimal goal. Ageing into ten-year age bands is feasible and I advocate using the strata 15–24, 25–34 and 45+, although some may wish to expand this slightly by having a further group of 45–54, the final group then comprising all those aged 55 years or more. Those under 15 years can be aged considerably more closely than this, but for the purposes of palaeoepidemiology such accuracy is most often redundant.[2]

It is of great importance to record the presence or absence of all the anatomical elements of the skeleton and the presence or absence of all the joints; when dealing with multicompartmental joints such as the elbow or knee, each compartment should receive individual attention. The need for such fastidiousness is that it is the total number of bones or joints which is likely to be the denominator for the estimation of prevalences and not the number of individuals.[3]

The next stage is the pathological examination and here the requirement is for the investigator to state clearly his criteria for making diagnoses or classifications; reference to an accepted authority is the least that is required. In a pitifully small number of cases it may be sufficient to note the presence of a pathognomonic sign, but when this cannot be done, and especially in cases which are likely to be controversial, the supporting evidence must be given. Remember that diagnosis in palaeopathology may be different from that in clinical practice or in radiology and that no palaeopathologist is likely somehow to diagnose conditions which present problems to the clinicians. From the epidemiological point of view it is safest to outline the operational criteria by which a case would be defined and it would be a happy state of affairs if operational criteria could be agreed for the major conditions likely to be found in the skeleton; as it is, few have been proposed and none to my knowledge has been universally agreed.

At this point it is a sound idea to construct plots of the age and sex distributions of the sample to see whether or not they conform to expectation. Unless it is a very special site—and this should be known in advance—the age distribution is likely to be roughly U-shaped, with a substantial number of juveniles but relatively few individuals in the 15–34 age range and an increasing number in succeeding age groups. The sex ratio should not differ greatly from unity. If the population distribution is markedly different from this, then one should consider if there is a good reason for it before venturing any further. In the absence of a good archaeological reason, then the most plausible explanation is that there were errors in the ageing and sexing; this explanation can be tested by repeating the estimations on a small random sample of the whole. If this seems to confirm that the original estimations were in error, you must decide whether the site is sufficiently important to warrant repeating the process on the entire population.

When you are satisfied with the preliminary data, age- and sex-specific prevalences for the common diseases can be calculated. The data (and the numbers on which they are based) should be included in a bone report and preferably in any papers published in the scientific press, although in the former they may have to appear in microfiche and in the latter not at all if space in the journal is at a premium. The age-specific prevalences of diseases which are known to be highly age related should be examined to ensure that the expected trend is present. For example, if the prevalence of osteoarthritis does *not* increase with age, then the ageing of the skeletons may be in error and must be checked. It is a *sine qua non* that the presence of conditions such as osteoarthritis must not be used as an ageing criterion otherwise epidemiological information will be lost.

For comparisons between populations the odds ratios of age-specific prevalences (or a common odds ratio) or direct standardisation should be used, preferably the former. If it is decided to use direct standardisation, the population which is used as the standard should be identified so that the numbers can be independently checked or used by other authors.

For the second kind of study, that is, where published data are to be compared, somewhat different constraints apply. First and foremost the investigator must satisfy himself that the data to be compared are truly compatible: that is, are the age classes and the diagnostic criteria the same in each; have prevalences been correctly calculated; and are the raw data given so that further calculations can be made? From what I know of the literature, it is more likely that the moon is made of green cheese than that all these requirements will be satisfied. Rather than turning to another field of study, the investigator should consider writing to the authors of the papers he would like to include in his analysis and ask whether the necessary data could be supplied. A courteous approach does sometimes produce the most unexpected results but the hit rate is not likely to be great and many authors may not reply, fearing the worst if their data should fall into the wrong hands. If you do propose to use another author's raw data then it is at least polite to suggest joint authorship of any publication which results; such a suggestion may not only show you as a considerate colleague but actually facilitate the release of the data to you.

At the time of writing this, the prospects of being able to carry out any comparative work on published material are slim and one of the purposes of writing this book is to encourage a discussion on the best way to record and report palaeopathological data and—sublime thought—perhaps arrive at a consensus; like Pindar's soul, we should exhaust the realm of the possible.[4]

NOTES

1. The results of such an exercise may not be very reassuring. In a study in which palaeopathologists were asked to diagnose osteoarthritis in a series of joints, the levels of agreement between observers on what we had supposed to be clear-cut examples gave us little encouragement to believe that it would ever be possible to compare data without adherence to very strict criteria. (T. Waldron and J. Rogers, Inter-observer variation in coding osteoarthritis in human skeletal remains, *International Journal of Osteoarchaeology*, 1991, 1, 49–56.

2. The methods used to age skeletons have come in for much criticism and the recent study in which estimated ages were compared with

true ages as shown on surviving coffin plates suggests that they are subject to considerable error (T. Molleson and M. Cox, *The Spitalfields project. Volume 2—The anthropology. The middling sort*, York, CBA, 1993, especially chapter 12). This is not the place to enter into a detailed critique of that study; suffice it to say that the design of the study was epidemiologically rather unsound and unless and until further and better designed studies come to the same conclusions as reported by Molleson and Cox, palaeopathologists need not be *too* disheartened.

3. For example, in the case of spondylolysis of the fifth lumbar vertebra, the denominator would be the total number of L5s; for fractures of the femur, the total number of femurs; for osteoarthritis of the elbow, the total number of elbows. If one is dealing with a disarticulated assemblage and wishing to calculate prevalences of disease, then the number of bones or joints is all that can be used, of course.

4. Pythian Odes, III, p 109.

8
A Question of Occupation

The quest to deduce as much as possible about the lives of individuals from their skeletons leads to some very extravagant claims being made about environmental stresses, parity, social status and occupation or occupationally related activities. In the case of occupation, such claims are made especially in relation to the presence of osteoarthritis. Faced with a skeleton with diseased joints or other abnormalities, some authors apparently cannot resist the urge to deduce an underlying cause and they frequently come up with the notion that the reason is to do with the individual's occupation, which they then confidently deduce on the basis of their observations and reasoning. Thus we may have sling throwers, weavers and corn grinders based on the presence of a bowed humerus and large muscle insertions, spinal deformities and osteoarthritis at the knees, spine and toes, respectively.[1] At the other extreme are those who consider that there is virtually nothing which can be gained from the examination of the skeleton, not always excluding age and sex. It is dull to suggest that the truth probably lies somewhere between these two extremes but there is no reason to suppose that the truth, when we know what it is, will always be interesting.

Were it really possible to be able to determine the occupation of past populations from the pathology in their skeletons this would be immensely useful and would be of great value to the palaeoepidemiologist. And because the prospect is so alluring, the premises which underpin this assumption are not always carefully examined;

if they are, then the proponents of the idea have not always wished to advertise the conclusions very widely.

Since osteoarthritis is the condition which is most frequently interpreted in the light of possible occupational or activity-related factors, I propose to consider now whether there is any basis for supposing that an occupation could, even under the most ideal circumstances, be derived from the pattern of osteoarthritis? Osteoarthritis is nowadays generally considered to be not so much a disease but rather the end result of (probably) a number of different processes and there are a number of factors known to affect the development of the condition. These include a genetic predisposition, sex, race, weight and movement.[2] Movement is of particular importance since the supposition which underlies the presumed relationship between work and osteoarthritis is that the changes occur in those joints which are most used or perhaps subject to repeated minor trauma as the result of forceful movement. There is no denying that movement is a crucial factor in the development of the changes in osteoarthritis, and joints which do not move, for whatever reason, do not get arthritic and so the idea has some apparent plausibility.

In all instances in which relationships are being inferred between, say, nutritional status and skeletal change, or life style and skeletal change, a reasonable starting point seems to me always to defer to what is known from modern clinical and epidemiological studies. In the case of occupational arthropathy there is a copious literature and a number of relationships have been proposed, many on the basis of case studies and cross-sectional studies. There is also an extremely voluminous literature on the relationship between what is often referred to as 'rheumatism' and occupation and on musculo-skeletal pain and occupation. It is important clearly to differentiate between osteoarthritis, rheumatism and musculo-skeletal pain in these studies. Unless otherwise specified, rheumatism in this context may be taken to mean soft tissue disease and not joint disease;[3] musculo-skeletal pain may be the product of both soft tissue and joint injury, but there is generally no means of knowing which is the major cause and so associations found between occupations and musculo-skeletal pain should not be considered to suggest a positive association with osteoarthritis. The results of studies which refer either to rheumatism or to musculo-skeletal pain are of no help to the palaeopathologist since it is not within his power to diagnose these in the skeleton. The only modern studies which are of help to the palaeoepidemiologist are those which specify osteoarthritis. In epidemiological as opposed to clinical studies, the presence of osteoarthritis depends upon the radiological demonstration of features such as joint space narrowing and the presence of osteophyte following the example set by Lawrence in his now classic studies.[4]

Many occupations have been found to have an excess of osteoarthritis at some joint or other compared with a control group and a few of these associations are shown in Table 8.1.[5] When examining the results of these studies it is worth bearing a few points in mind. Firstly, there is very little consistency about the results; for example, some authors find that coal miners have a high prevalence of osteoarthritis of the spine whereas others do not, that there are many negative studies in which *no* association is found between work and osteoarthritis,[6] that many people who work in strenuous occupations do not get osteoarthritis of any joint and, finally, that many people who work in sedentary occupations or who do not work at all nevertheless do develop osteoarthritis. Probably the best demonstrated relationships are those which Hadler and his colleagues found between the disposition of osteoarthritis of the hands and the tasks being undertaken by women in a worsted mill in Virginia in the USA.[7] The women in the mill were engaged in three tasks: spinning, burling and windings. In all three groups the right (dominant) hand was more affected than the left but the winders were much less likely to have osteoarthritis in the second and third digits than burlers or spinners whilst the spinners alone had no involvement of the fifth digit.

A more recent study has shown an impressive relationship between farming and osteoarthritis of the hip, farmers having an odds ratio of approximately 9 compared with the general population.[8]

The inescapable impression which one gets from a review of the available literature, however, is that there is no convincing evidence of a *consistent* relationship between a particular occupation and a particular form of osteoarthritis and, given the multifactorial nature

Table 8.1   Some reported associations between occupation and osteoarthritis

Site(s)	Occupation
Foot, knee	Ballet dancers
Wrist, elbow	Chipping and grinding operators
	Foundry workers
Metacarpo-phalangeal joints	Jackhammer operators
Knee	Labourers
Spine, knee	Miners
Hand	Mill workers
Hip	Farmers

Data from several sources.

of the condition, this is probably what one ought to expect. Perhaps the most which can be said is that in some occupations in which repetitive and strenuous movements of a few joints occurs, this movement will determine which joints are affected in those predisposed to the disease.

To judge from modern epidemiological work then, I suggest there is very little reason to assume that occupation is related to osteoarthritis in any consistent or coherent manner, but let us suppose that it was; under those circumstances would we be able to infer an occupation from the pattern of osteoarthritis: that is, can we argue from the effects we see in the bone to the ultimate cause?

We must first begin by considering some of the possibilities about the cause of osteoarthritis and there seem to me to be three, which we could call the simple, plural and complex models. The simple model (Figure 8.1a) assumes that there is only one cause of the disease; the plural model (Figure 8.1b) assumes that there are many causes but that they act independently of each other; finally the complex model also assumes that there are many causes but in this case they must all act together (Figure 8.1c).[9] It would be possible—at least in theory—for a modern epidemiologist, using a variety of methods, to make a reasonable attempt to establish which of the models most closely accorded with his observations.

What is equally clear is that the palaeoepidemiologist, starting with the effect and trying to argue back to cause, could succeed *only* if the simple model prevailed (Figure 8.2). That is to say, the

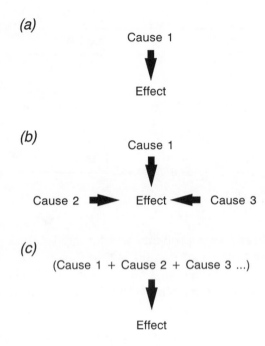

Figure 8.1 Models of different causes of osteoarthritis. (a) Simple model, with only a single cause; (b) plural model with several causes but each acting independently and (c) complex model with several causes all of which need to act together

cause of osteoarthritis could only be inferred if it were known that it had only a single cause. In the plural model, it would be impossible to say with any confidence—probably even with any reason—which of the many causes was operating in a single case. Similarly, in the complex model, no inference could be made about which of the many causes, which needed to be acting together, was having the predominant effect, if indeed it could be said that *any* was predominant.

Since we know that occupation is *not* the sole cause of osteoarthritis, there cannot be any likelihood of being able to deduce the former from the latter. And there is another matter which is also acting against being able to do so. Even in those cases where occupationally related activity does seem to be an important determinant in the expression of osteoarthritis, there are no unique features about this expression. Osteoarthritis of the hands

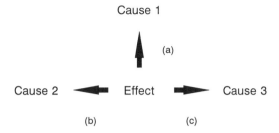

(a) Simple model

(a) or (b) or (c) Plural model

(a+b+c) Complex model

Figure 8.2   Model relating an effect (osteoarthritis) back to its cause (or causes). It will be clear that if a single cause is sought, then this will only be possible following the simple model in Figure 8.1a, that is, if there is only one cause

is not exclusive to worsted mill workers nor osteoarthritis of the hip to farmers; the vast majority of individuals who develop osteoarthritis at these sites are not in these occupations, perhaps in no occupation at all. Given a skeleton with osteoarthritis of the hip, and given that we believe that farmers have a substantial predisposition to develop the disease here—a relative risk of 9, let us say—this still leaves us unable to say whether the skeleton before us was that of a farmer or any one of the thousands of non-farmers who might have had it. We could, of course, be right; it *might* be the farmer, but we would be right for the wrong reason.

The only way in which an occupation could accurately be determined in a single skeleton would be if the appearance of the disease at a single site, or a specific combination of sites, was unique to those following a single occupation. And we know that this is not the case.

There is a somewhat better prospect of being able to infer something about activity in populations from the basis of their osteoarthritis. For example let us suppose that in one population there was a predominance of osteoarthritis at the hand, shoulder and knee, whereas in another, separated perhaps by a considerable

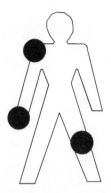 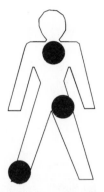

Figure 8.3 Diagram to show the distribution of osteoarthritis in two hypothetical populations. In the first (on the left), the disease occurs predominantly in the hand, shoulder and knee, whereas in the second (on the right), the sterno-clavicular joint, hip and foot are mainly affected. If it were known that the two populations pursued different activities, this might be one explanation for the differences seen

interval of time from the first, the major sites affected were the sterno-clavicular joint, hip and foot, then clearly different factors are likely to be operating in the two to produce these distinct patterns of disease (Figure 8.3). There would be many factors to consider, activity being one, and if, from other evidence, it were known that the ways of life were greatly different—one being an urban group and one mainly agricultural—then it would be permissible to speculate on the extent to which the varying activities undertaken by each group might account for the distribution of the osteoarthritis. If we were to conclude that farming activities somehow contributed to the greater prevalence of osteoarthritis of the hip in the second population, this would still not allow us to pick out the farmers from the group on the basis of them having osteoarthritis for the reasons given above.[10]

This brief sketch will, I hope, act to deter some of the more extravagant claims which are made about the ability to deduce occupation from the skeleton, although I cannot be overly optimistic. There is a perfectly understandable drive to make the most of what little evidence survives in the skeleton and this sometimes has the effect of overwhelming the critical faculties. It would be possible to point to other examples where too much may be being made of too little, or where interpretation is outstripping hard evidence, and it generally happens in areas where there is little

clinical evidence to back up the suppositions or where the observers have not troubled to make themselves aware of what there
is. The words of Thomas McKeown are very germane in this
context. He wrote

> In general ... I am doubtful about the reliability of much historical evidence
> related to health, unless it has been screened critically through present-day
> experience.[11]

The same is true for palaeopathological evidence, and those who
work in this field ignore McKeown's caveat at their peril.

NOTES

1. These examples, which are not suggested as being the most extreme,
    were proposed by J. Cameron, *The skeleton on British neolithic man*,
    London, Williams and Norgate, 1934, pp 209–22; C. Wells, Weaver,
    tailor or shoemaker? An osteological detective story, *Medical and
    Biological Illustration*, 1967, 17, 39–47; and T. Molleson, Seed prepara-
    tion in the Mesolithic: the osteological evidence, *Antiquity*, 1989, 63,
    356–62.
2. P.A. Dieppe, Osteoarthritis. A review, *Journal of the Royal College of
    Physicians of London*, 1990, 24, 262–7.
3. For a review of soft tissue rheumatism and occupation (albeit some-
    what dated now), see J.A.D. Anderson, Rheumatism in industry: a
    review, *British Journal of Industrial Medicine*, 1971, 28, 103–21.
4. Lawrence published many studies on the epidemiology of osteoarth-
    ritis and the relationship with occupation. His results are sum-
    marised in J.S. Lawrence, *Rheumatism in populations*, London,
    Heinemann Medical Books, 1977; this book contains references to the
    original papers and is an excellent source if it is wished to consult
    them. He and his colleagues also undertook a number of cross-sec-
    tional studies of general population samples, taking X-rays of many
    joints. It is probably true to say that studies such as his, requiring
    much exposure to X-rays by normal subjects, would not be permitted
    nowadays with our much stricter control of X-ray exposure and it is
    very unlikely that Lawrence's studies will be repeated or extended.
5. For a much more comprehensive list the reader if referred to K.A.R.
    Kennedy's table in his chapter, Skeletal markers of occupational
    stress, In: *Reconstruction of life from the skeleton*, edited by M.Y. Iscan
    and K.A.R. Kennedy, New York, Alan Liss, 1989, pp 129–60. The table

takes up no less than 15 pages and is a list which repays study if only for the completely uncritical way in which the data are presented and the total lack of discrimination shown.

6. It is generally more difficult to have a paper with negative results published than one with positive results and this leads to a certain amount of publication bias; in any discipline there will always be found more papers with positive than negative findings. This bias assumes some importance when reviews are undertaken and where the strength of an association may be deduced by balancing the number of positive and negative results; in any such process, the positive will outweigh the negatives. The same considerations also apply when a statistical review—a so-called meta-analysis—is being undertaken of published data.

7. Hadler's observations are contained in two excellent papers and are further summarised in a chapter in a book; all three are worth consulting. N.M. Hadler, Industrial rheumatology. Clinical investigations into the influence of the pattern of usage on the pattern of regional musculoskeletal disease, *Arthritis and Rheumatism*, 1977, 20, 1019–25; N.M. Hadler, D.B. Gillings, H.R. Imbus, P.M. Levitin, D. Makuc, P.D. Utsinger, W.J. Yount, D. Slusser and N. Moskovitz, Hand structure and function in an industrial setting. Influence of three patterns of stereotyped repetitive usage, *Arthritis and Rheumatism*, 1978, 21, 210–20; N.M. Hadler, The variable of usage in the epidemiology of osteoarthris, In: *Epidemiology or osteoarthritis*, edited by J.G. Peyron, London, Geigy, 1980, pp 164–71.

8. P. Croft, D. Coggon, M. Cruddas and C. Cooper, Osteoarthritis of the hip: an occupational disease in farmers, *British Medical Journal*, 1992, 304, 1269–72. The odds ratio was 9.3 with a 95% CI of 1.9–44.5. The increased risk did not seem to be attributed with any particular type of farming and it was suggested that heavy lifting was the most likely explanation. This study confirmed the results of an earlier investigation by the same group in which mechanical overloading of the hip was again blamed for the excess of this disease in farmers (P. Croft, C. Cooper, C. Wickham and D. Coggon, Osteoarthritis of the hip and occupational activity, *Scandinavian Journal of Work, Environment and Health*, 1992, 18, 59–63).

9. Note that we are considering here *possibilities* and not actualities; no-one seriously doubts now that osteoarthritis has a multifactorial aetiology; the models proposed in this section are merely to illustrate the argument that follows.

10. Whether osteoarthritis is the best marker to use for deducing patterns of activity in a population is by no means certain but this is not the place to enter into that discussion. Suffice it to say that the pattern of

enthesophytes may be more sensitive since—in the absence of some other diseases—these occur at tendon insertions which have been subjected to the trauma consequent upon continual wear and tear. The pattern of enthesophytes with populations may provide better evidence of activity than osteoarthritis and some attempts have been made in this direction; see, for example, O. Dutour, Enthesopathies (lesions of muscular insertions) as indicators of the activities of neolithic Saharan populations, *American Journal of Physical Anthropology*, 1986, 71, 221–4.

11. T. McKeown, *The origins of human disease*, Oxford, Blackwell, 1988, p 10.

Last Words

Palaeopathology has given me—and gives to many others—a great deal of pleasure and that in itself is sufficient reason to pursue it. There is a greater, deeper source of satisfaction, however, and that is in knowing that, to whatever small degree, one is adding to the knowledge and understanding of our ancestors; we might also be able to contribute to an understanding of the natural history of disease and this may have relevance to those who only study medicine in a modern context. If we intend our study to have the latter purpose, more stringent criteria are required in the interpretation and presentation of our observations; it is hoped that the ideas set out in this book will help some towards this.

Some readers may object that the emphasis throughout has been too restrictive with too little allowance made for interpretation; they may perhaps say with Sydney Smith (the pathologist, not the cleric) that 'My report was partly speculative ... but without speculation it would not have been much use.'[1] And, of course, it is idle—even perverse—to suggest that one can advance any subject without interpretation and speculation. Writing about the role of the historian, Isaiah Berlin reminds us: 'That to exercise their proper function [they] require the capacity for imaginative insight, without which the bones of the past remain dry and lifeless. To deploy it is, and always has been, a risky business'.[2] It is the risks attached to imaginative insight which I am anxious to point out; interpretation and speculation are fine so long as their bounds are confined by the limits of the observations upon which they are based and by our own experience and that of others, who are perhaps wiser than we. Let me close with Isaiah Berlin again: in his essay on Vico, who was one of the most original thinkers of the 18th century, he writes: 'The crucial role he [Vico] assigns to the imagination must not blind us—and did not blind him—to the necessity for verification; he allows that critical methods of examining evidence are indispensable'.[3]

Critical methods for examining evidence are no less dispensable in palaeopathology than in any other field of serious human endeavour.

NOTES

1. S. Smith, *Mostly murder*, London, Harrap, 1959, p 15.
2. I. Berlin, Giambattista Vico and cultural history, In: *The crooked timber of humanity*, London, Fontana Press, 1991, p 69.
3. Berlin, *op cit*, p 64.

Index